Melody of Mind

Melody of Mind

Fakir Mohan Sahoo

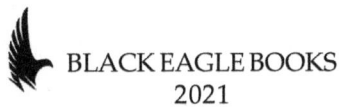
BLACK EAGLE BOOKS
2021

BLACK EAGLE BOOKS

USA address:
7464 Wisdom Lane
Dublin, OH 43016

India address:
E/312, Trident Galaxy, Kalinga Nagar,
Bhubaneswar-751003, Odisha, India

E-mail: info@blackeaglebooks.org
Website: www.blackeaglebooks.org

First International Edition Published by
BLACK EAGLE BOOKS, 2021

MELODY OF MIND
by Fakir Mohan Sahoo

Original Copyright © **Fakir Mohan Sahoo**

All rights reserved. No part of this publication may be reproduced, stored in a retrieval system, or transmitted, in any form or by any means, electronic, mechanical, photocopying, recording or otherwise without the prior permission of the publisher.

Cover & Interior Design: Ezy's Publication

ISBN- 978-1-64560-213-2 (Paperback)
Library of Congress Control Number: 2021946517

Printed in United States of America

To,
Mr. Ashok Kumar Mohapatra
for bonding us with beauties
of his friendliness

Books by the Author

- Cognitive styles & interpersonal behaviour
- Affective sensitivity & cognitive styles
- Psychology in Indian context (Edited)
- Environment & behaviour
- Child rearing & educating assistance manual
- Dynamics of human helplessness
- Sex roles in transition
- Behavioural issues in ageing (Edited)
- Atlas of mind
- Mysteries of mind
- Wonders of mind
- Splendours of mind
- Mind management
- Tools of mind
- Landscape of mind
- Plasticity of mind
- Happiness flows

Books in Odia

- Bichitra mana
- Manasika bikruti
- Jiban prabahare manasika bikruti
- Adhuni ka jibanare manasika chapa
- Manara manachitra
- Manastatvika bikasare saisaba parba
- Byaktitva & netrutva
- Nari manastatva
- Manastatvika bikasara godhuli parba
- Sisu manara bigyan
- Sachitra mana
- Sabala mana, saphala jibana
- Manastatvika bikasara balya parba
- Manastatvika bikasara kaishore parba
- Manasika samasya O samadhan
- Manara rahasya
- Sukhanubhutira marmakatha
- Jibana O' manastatwa
- Tallinata
- Sahitya O' manastatwa
- Chapamukta jeeban
- Sakshyatakara
- Manastatwika bikashar jouban parba
- Sukhanubhutira marmakatha

Preface

The book "Melody of Mind" is floated at a time when the world is afflicted by fear psychosis. The sickening events caused by COVID 19 are overpowering our life transactions. The agonizing news in the media, saddening stories of people, and the loss of human lives have created a climate of collective depression. Although experts of different persuasions have joined hands to find out a protective umbrella, the hope and aspiration has not yet taken a tangible reality.

As an applied science of mind management, psychology is offering some mental fighters. Since internal protectors are at least as important as external protectors, the counselling tips appear to be immensely valuable. Fortunately, many of such psychological aids are very much consistent with our Indic scholarship and indigenous wisdom (e.g., spirituality and meditation). The book is an attempt in the direction of educating and elevating psychological resources within.

I wish to thank Mr. Ashok K. Parida and Ashis K. Mohanty for their assistance in the process of publication. I am happy to record my appreciation to Ms. Sangeeta S. Barla for arranging the materials. I am greatly appreciative of the gestures of Dr. Satya Pattnaik (Ohio, USA) for initiating a friendly and valuable publication relationship.

July 24, 2021   **F.M. Sahoo**
Sai Chhaya
VIM 99, Sailashree Vihar
Bhubaneswar 751021 India
Tele 91 9437121279 (M)

CONTENTS

Increasing Happiness in Your Life	11
Preventing the Bad	14
Promoting the Good	22
Seven Ways for Combating Depression	28
Performance Excellence	31
The Second Brain in the Gut	34
Genes Are Not Destiny	38
Adding Life to Years	45
Awareness of Death	51
Value Education	58
Avoiding Overthinking	69
Attitude of Gratitude	74
Childhood Antecedents of Self-Efficacy	79
Flow: Mechanism of Living in the Present	86
Savouring: An Alternative for Living in the Present	91
Preventing Negative Changes Related to Aging	96
Social Brain	99
Storytelling: The Style that Works in Leadership Talks	102
What's Ahead	104
Gratitude	108
Expanding the Contours of Pleasure	113
Living a Pleasurable Life	117
Building Flourishing Relationship	122
Positive Life Events	129
Spirituality	132
The Buffering Role of Humour	135
Positive Moods and Immune Functioning	141
Skills to Manage Fear in an Unsafe World	145
How to Control Your Anger	151
Meditation	156
Building Psychological Resilience	159
Pandemic and Rebuilding of Life	171
Finding Silver Lining in a Cloud	178

Increasing Happiness in Your Life

While there are numerous theories of happiness and countless happiness-boosting techniques, people harbor questions relating to their feasibility. Is it possible to comply with all the suggestions to make myself happier? David Myers (1993), an expert on the subject and author of the book *"The Pursuit of Happiness"* provides general strategies for increasing happiness in your life. Have a close look and translate them into your daily habits.

- Realize that enduring happiness doesn't come from success. People adapt to changing circumstances – even to wealth or a disability. Thus, wealth is like health; its utter absence breeds misery, but having it (or any circumstance we long for) doesn't guarantee happiness.
- Take control of your time. Happy people feel in control of their lives, often aided by mastering their use of time. It helps to set goals and break them into daily aims. Although we often overestimate how much we will accomplish in any given day (leaving us frustrated), we generally underestimate how much we will accomplish in a year, given just a little progress every day.
- Act happy. We can sometimes act ourselves into a frame of mind. Manipulated into a smiling expression,

people feel better; when they scowl, the whole world seems to scowl back. So put on a happy face. Talk, as if you feel positive self-esteem, are optimistic, and are outgoing. Going through the motions can trigger the emotions.

- Seek work and leisure that engages your skills. Happy people often are in a zone called "flow" – absorbed in a task that challenges them without overwhelming them. The most expensive forms of leisure (sitting on a yacht) often provide less flow experiences than gardening, socializing, or craft work.
- Join the "movement"movement. An avalanche of research reveals that aerobic exercises not only promote health and energy, it is also an antidote to mild depression and anxiety. Sound minds reside in sound bodies.
- Give your body the sleep it wants. Happy people live active vigorous lives, yet reserve time for renewing sleep and solitude. Many people suffer from a sleep debt, with resulting fatigue, diminished alertness, and gloomy moods.
- Give priority to close relationships. Intimate friendship with those who care deeply about you can help you weather difficult times. Confiding is good for soul and body. Resolve to nurture your closest relationships, to not take those closest to you for granted, to display to them the sort of kindness that you display to others, to affirm them, to play together and share together. To rejuvenate your affections, resolve in such ways to act lovingly.
- Focus beyond the self. Reach out to those in need. Happiness increases helpfulness (those who feel good do good). But doing good also makes one feel good.

- Keep a gratitude journal. Those who pause each day to reflect on some positive aspects of their lives (their health, friends, family, freedom, education, natural surroundings and so on) experience heightened well-being.
- Nurture your spiritual self. For many people, faith provides a support community, a reason to focus beyond self and a sense of purpose and hope. A bulk of studies finds that actively religious people are happier and that they cope better with crises.

■

Preventing the Bad

Prevention is better than cure. This conventional wisdom is applicable to many domains of human life including mental health. The process of stopping the bad involves efforts to prevent negative things from occurring later, and it can be divided into primary and secondary prevention. **Primary prevention** lessens or eliminates physical or psychological problems *before* they appear. **Secondary prevention** lessens or eliminates problems *after* they have appeared.

As indicated, primary intervention reflects actions that people take to lessen or remove the likelihood of subsequent psychological difficulties or physical problems. With primary prevention, people are not yet manifesting any problems, and it is only later that such problems will appear if protective, or prophylactic steps are not taken. When primary prevention is aimed at entire community it is called **universal prevention** (e.g., Childhood immunization). When it is focused on a particular at-risk population, it is called **selective prevention** (mid-day meals to reduce possible drop-outs in schools).

For each of these primary and secondary approaches, the following constitutes the slogan

    Primary Prevention: "Stop the bad before it happens"

    Secondary Prevention: "Fix the Problem"

Primary prevention activities are based on hope for the future. Primary prevention sometimes may occur at the governmental level. By setting and enforcing laws that allow people to succeed because of their merits and efforts, a government can lessen subsequent negative consequences for its citizens. For example, with legislation against drunk drivers, roadside accidents can be reduced. Similarly, laws prohibiting discrimination can reduce the possibilities of racial and social violence.

On the whole, primary preventions are quite effective. Psychologists have examined the effectiveness of prevention programmes on children's and adolescents' behavioural and social problems. They found that the prevention programmes are effective in reducing problems.

Psychologists have offered suggestions for implementing successful primary preventions. First, the targeted populations should be given knowledge about the risky behaviour to be prevented. Second, the programme should be attractive. It should motivate potential participants to increase the desirable behaviour and decrease the undesirable ones. The programme should teach problem solving skills as well as how to resist regressing into previous counter-productive pattern. Finally, data should be gathered to enable evaluation of the programme's accomplishment.

Primary Prevention for Children

Several primary preventions target at-risk children and youth. It is useful to teach problem solving skills to children who are likely to use inappropriate, impulsive responses when encountering interpersonal problems. Such children are projected to have unhappy lives in which they would resort to crime and aggressive behaviour. As an antidote to these predicted problems, the children are taught to come up with ways, other than aggressive outbursts, to reach their goals. These successful primary prevention programmes have been expanded to middle schools.

A prevention programme in helping children at risk for depression has been found to be successful. Using Seligman's learned optimism model, children's attribution (explanatory styles) may be identified. It is important to note that children employing internal (I am responsible) permanent and global (pervading to all areas of life) attributions are considered helpless and vulnerable to depression. A 12-week programme may be undertaken where children are counseled to use external (other factors are also responsible for the bad event), temporary and specific (only a single area of my life is affected) attribution to explain bad (negative) events. It is found that the group receiving such prevention package shows considerable improvement in their optimistic outlook.

Primary Prevention for the Elderly

Prevention programmes for the elderly can focus on many different objectives including screening to lessen the probability of later physical health problems and diseases, checking living arrangements to remove physical hazards that can lead to falls and other accidents and attempts to maximize the elders' work, social and interpersonal engagements. One such intriguing prevention programmes, called **Grandma Please**, involves grandchildren who telephone their grandparents after school. The programme is based on compelling premise that keeping the elderly involved and actively participating in their families prevent them from spiraling into lives of isolation and depression.

Secondary Prevention

Secondary prevention addresses a problem as it begins to unfold. Compared to primary prevention, secondary prevention occurs later in the temporal sequence of the unfolding problem. Snyder described secondary prevention as occurring when the individual produces thoughts or actions to eliminate, reduce, or contain the problem once it appeared. Therefore, time in relation to the problem is a key differentiating factor in these two types of prevention, with primary prevention involving actions initiated before a problem has developed, and secondary prevention involving actions taken after the problem has appeared.

Secondary prevention is synonymous with psychotherapy. Although most people realize that there are numerous forms of psychotherapies, it may surprise many to learn that helpers presently are using more than 400 forms of psychotherapies.

We view psychotherapy as a prime example of secondary prevention because people who come for such treatment know that they have specific problems that are beyond their capabilities to handle, and this is what leads them to obtain help. The specific problems and life stressors trigger the seeking of psychological assistance. Of course, when psychotherapy is successful, it also may produce the primary prevention characteristics of lessening or preventing recurrence of similar problems in the future.

From the earliest summaries of the effectiveness of psychotherapies to more contemporary ones, there is consistent evidence that psychotherapy improves the lives of adults and children. When we say that psychotherapy "works" we mean than there is a lessening of the severity and/or frequency of the client's problem and symptoms. On an average, a person who has undergone psychotherapy has improved by a magnitude of 1 standard deviation (that is, she or he is about 34% better off) on various outcome markers, relative to the person who has not undergone psychotherapy. Furthermore, persons who have undergone psychotherapy intervention report being very satisfied with their experience.

It is believed that hope is the underlying principle common to all successful psychotherapy approaches. Placebo effects in psychotherapy represent how much clients will improve if they are motivated to believe that change will happen.

Most psychotherapy approaches have used "problem talk" rather than "solution talk". This is to say the traditional focus has been on decreasing negative thoughts and behaviours rather than building of positive thoughts and behaviours. Even though pathology approach to thinking about human behaviour still is the prevailing model, in recent years many therapists have begun to attend to clients' strength. Likewise, a client sometimes must unlearn negative thoughts and behaviours before learning positive ones.

Self-Management

Prior to indicating the approach of positive psychology, it is useful to outline effective lessening of problems through self-management.

One such is Bandura's *self-efficacy model*. According to this model, a client can learn efficacy beliefs through (1) actual performance accomplishment in the problem area, (2) modeling another person who is coping effectively, (3) verbal persuasion by the helper, and (4) controlling negative cognitive process by learning to implement positive moods. It is important to note that there are specific target problems in such self-efficacy approaches.

A second type of self-management involves Meichenbaum's (1977) *self-instructional training*. It is typically aimed at the problem of anxiety. The initial stage of this approach is gathering information about the problem including maladaptive cognitions. This is accomplished when the helper asks the client to imagine the problem and then describe the ongoing internal dialogue. In the second stage of Meichwnbaum's treatment approach, the client is taught more adaptive internal dialogues. Lastly the client practices these new coping dialogues in order to strengthen the likelihood of actually using them.

A third self-management approach is Kanfer's *three-stage self-management model*. In the first stage, self-monitoring, the client observes the problematic behaviour in the context of its antecedents and consequences. In the second stage, self-evaluation, the client learns to compare the ongoing problematic behaviour with the desired improved standard of performance and realizes that she or he is falling below the standard. In the third stage, self-reinforcement, the client learns to reinforce him or herself (with rewards and punishments) for controlling the undesired behaviour. Additionally, the client must be committed to change.

Positive Psychology Approach

Positive psychology approaches emphasize positive parameters in the change process. Although there are various forms of using this approach in helping process, two model techniques may be indicated here.

Seligman's *learned optimism model* has been extensively used. According to Seligman, explaining bad (negative) events in internal (personal), stable and global terms is maladaptive, whereas explaining these events with external, unstable (temporary) and specific terms is adaptive. In contrast, explaining good (positive) events with personal, permanent and pervasive terms is adaptive whereas using external, unstable and specific attributions is unhealthy.

Hence, the main role of the helper involves reattribution training. If the client is using maladaptive attributions, the helper may train the client to change from maladaptive to adaptive explanatory style. An example may illustrate the point. For example, a person is experiencing helplessness (depression) because of an antecedent of adversity.

Adversity: Ravi fails the exam
Belief: I am worthless
Consequence: I feel depressed

In this typical case, the helper has to **dispute** the belief. **Disputation** can be effected through persuasion (that Ravi is not worthless) or confrontation (by providing evidence of success in various domains). Once the faulty belief (that Ravi is worthless) is dispelled, Ravi may regain **energization**. Thus, ABCDE (Antecedent Belief Consequence Disputation Energization) model works as an effective strategy.

In addition to learned optimism therapy, some attention has been given to implementing what has been called **hope therapy**. Two parameters important in hope theory include goals and pathways. Accordingly, clients are helped to identify their goals, understand their goals and spell out their commitment. They are also helped to delineate pathways for attainment of their goals. A number of studies have found that hope intervention works better than **reminiscence therapy** where participants recall their pleasurable times. Hope therapy has been employed extensively to address the problems of passivity and depression in the elderly.

In essence, positive psychology approach involves the processes to accentuate clients' strength. Attempts are directed to make clients more productive and happier. Obviously such processes eliminate or attenuate problem behaviours. In positive psychology version, this is termed **wellness-therapy**.

Promoting the Good

There are two broad approaches to the objective of promoting the good. The first view is hedonic well-being in maximizing pleasurable experiences. The second view, called eudaimonic perspective, stresses goals and meaningfulness. **Primary enhancement** involves the efforts to establish optimal functioning and happiness. As shown by the Figure indicated below, primary enhancement involves attempts either to increase hedonic well-being by increasing pleasurable moments or by augmenting eudaimonic well-being by setting goals and reaching goals. Whereas hedonic primary enhancements tap indulgence in pleasure and satisfaction of appetites and needs, eudaimonic primary enhancement emphasize effective functioning and happiness as a desirable result of the goal pursuit process. In this regard, it should be noted that there is a clear distinction between hedonic and eudaimonic human needs.

Primary Enhancement	Secondary Enhancement
Establish optimal functioning & satisfaction	Sustain and build upon already optimal functioning & satisfaction

In an evolutionary sense, particular activities are biologically predisposed to produce satisfaction. An evolutionary premise is that people experience pleasure under the circumstances favourable to the propagation of the human species. Accordingly, happiness results from close interpersonal ties, especially those that lead to mating and protection of the offspring.

Primary Enhancement and Psychological Health

Many people in their death beds may think, "I wish I had spent more time with my family". This suggests that our relationships are crucial for life satisfaction. Indeed, for most people, interpersonal relationship with lovers, family and good friends provide the most powerful sources of well-being and life satisfaction.

Engaging in shared activities that are enjoyable enhances psychological well-being, especially if such joint participation entails arousing and novel activities. Likewise, it is beneficial for couples to tackle intrinsically motivated activities in which they can share aspects of their lives and become absorbed in the ongoing flow of their behaviours.

Beyond the relationship with one's mate, primary enhancement satisfactions also can come from other relationships, such as family and friends. Arranging living circumstances within close physical proximity to kin also can produce the social supports that are crucial for happiness. So too, can the close network of a few friends produce contentment.

Another relationship that produces happiness is involvement in religion and spiritual matters. In part, this may reflect the fact that religiosity and prayer are related to higher hope. Religious faith and various other religious practices can be predictive of hope and optimism. Likewise, some of the satisfaction from religions probably stems from the social contacts it provides. Happiness also may result from the spirituality stemming with a higher power. On this point, there is accruing scientific evidence of a possible genetic link to human spirituality needs.

Gainful **employment** also is an important source of happiness. To the degree people are satisfied with their work, they also are happier (An overall correlation of .40 between being employed and level of happiness). The reason for this finding is that, for many people, work provides a social network and it also allows for the testing of talents and skills.

Leisure activities can also bring pleasure. Relaxing, resting, and eating a good meal will have the short-term effect of making people feel better. Recreational activities such as sports, dancing and listening to music allow people to make life enjoyable.

Whatever the particular primary enhancement activities may be, those activities that are totally absorbing are the most enjoyable. Csikszentmihalyi and his colleagues have studied circumstance that lead to a sense of total engagement. Such activities typically are intrinsically fascinating, and they stretch talents to satisfying levels. This type of primary enhancement is called **flow experience**, and artists, surgeons, writers, and other professionals report such flow in their work.

Yet another route to attaining a series of contentment is through **here-and-now contemplation** of one's external and internal environment. Indeed, a common thread in Eastern thought is that immense pleasure is to be attained through "being" or experiencing. Even in Western societies, meditation upon internal experiences or thought has gained many followers. **Meditation** has been defined as a "family of techniques which have" a common conscious attempt to focus attention in a nonanalytic way, and an attempt not to dwell on discursive, ruminating thought. For example, mindfulness meditation involves a nonjudgmental attention that allows a sense of peacefulness, serenity, and pleasure. Seven qualities of mindfulness meditation include: nonjudging, acceptance, openness, nonstriving, patience, trust, and letting go. Likewise, in what is called **concentrative meditation**, awareness is restricted by focusing on a thought or object such as a personal mantra, breath, or word.

Another process that is meditation like in its operation is savouring. **Savouring** involves thoughts or actions that are aimed at appreciating and perhaps amplifying a positive experience of some sort. According to Fred Bryant (2005), who is the psychologist who coined the term, savouring can take three temporal forms:
- Anticipation or enjoyment of forthcoming positive event
- Being in the moment, or thinking and doing things to intensify and perhaps prolong a positive event as it occurs
- Reminiscing or looking back at a positive event to rekindle the favourable feeling or thought

Furthermore, savouring can take the following forms:
- Sharing with others
- Taking "mental photographs" to build one's memories
- Congratulating oneself
- Comparing with what one has felt in other circumstances
- Sharpening senses through concentration
- Becoming absorbed in the moment
- Expressing oneself through behaviour (laughing, shouting, pumping one's fist in the air)
- Realizing how fleeting and precious the experience is

- Counting one's blessings

There is yet more that people can do beyond savouring. Psychologist Barbara Fredrickson has shown that experience of positive emotion builds internal resources and expands the contours of activity. Negative emotion, in contrast, limits the scope of activity. Positive emotions can be induced by listening to a favorite piece of music or by watching a good movie.

Psychologist Ilardi and his colleagues at the University of Kansas have initiated a new treatment for the prevention of depression, and the enhancement of personal happiness. It is called **Therapeutic Lifestyle Change (TLC)**. The basic tanet of TLC is that engaging in certain approach to one's lifestyle, especially those activities that were natural parts of the lives of our ancestors.

The following components constitute TLC:
- Exercise (35 mts at-least thrice a week)
- Omega3 fatty acid supplement
- Exposure of light (30 mts bright sunlight per day)
- Stop rumination (call friends)
- At least 7/8 hours of sleep every night
- Social contact

Secondary Enhancement

Secondary enhancement of psychological health enables people to maximize their pleasure by building on their pre-existing positive mental health. Past psychological moments often involve important human connections, such as the birth of a child, a wedding, the graduation of a loved one.

The existentialist contemplation of the meaning in life is yet another approach to achieving a transcendently gratifying experience. Viktor Frankl considering the question: What is the nature of meaning in life? He concluded that the ultimate life meaning comes from thinking about our goals and purposes. Furthermore, he speculated that the ultimate satisfaction comes from contemplating our purpose during times in which we are suffering.

Another transcending experience involves seeing another person doing something that is so special that it is awe-inspiring or elevating.

Seven Ways for Combating Depression

Depression is comparable to the problem of cough and cold in our day-to-day lives. Over the decades it has become more rampant and bothering. How can we handle it so that we would live in peace and prosperity. It is challenging; yet we can handle it. It is said: *Birds of depression may fly over our heads, but we must not allow these birds to build their nests in our heads.* Here is some advice from psychological research.

1. Use optimistic explanatory styles. Accidents do happen in the best regulated families. When bad (negative) events do happen, people generally ask three questions: Who is responsible? How long would its effects stay? How pervasive would be its effect? People blaming themselves as the sole cause for the bad events feel highly depressed. People considering the effect as permanent and pervasive also feel dejected. So analyze *external* causes for the bad events and treat the negative events as temporary and specific (If it has happened in the social area, keep it confined to the social domain; if it has happened in professional sector, keep it limited to professional area). If positive (good) events happen, explain in terms of personal, permanent and pervasive factors. This will reduce your depression and augment your happiness.

2. Do not make unfavourable comparisons. Many people compare themselves with the rich, powerful and the highly placed and feel depressed. Think of the underprivileged and the downtrodden. Of several forms of Buddhist meditation, *compassion meditation* is a major form. People are trained to mediate and think of the people in plight. A magnificent Chinese proverb says: A man was complaining of his shoes till he came across a person without a leg.

3. Pursue intentional activities. A major form of behavioural mechanism for combating depression involves intentional activities such as hobbies. A self-set task takes away depression. Develop and pursue hobbies. Introduce elements of variety into your intentional activities. If you are taking a morning walk every day, do not start from the same point or at the specific time every day. Be flexible. Start 15 minutes earlier or later. Similarly change your route. Do not have a mechanical way of completing your task. This is not a task; it is a pleasurable activity for you.

4. Adopt instrumental coping, not ruminating coping. When confronted with coping problems, a number of individuals adopt ruminating strategy. They spend a lot of time analyzing the cause of the problem. Analysis is sometimes paralysis. There is consistent research finding that women use *ruminating coping* while men employ *instrumental coping*. For dealing with depression, use instrumental coping. Do whatever can be done best. Doing doable things would help you to tide over the situation.

5. Define difficult situations as challenging but controllable, never see them as threatening. If you see a snake and run, you get into fear. If you see a snake and hit it with a stick you get into anger. What would determine your emotion is the way you define the situation. If you define it threatening, you would be crippled. If you define it challenging, your efforts would be augmented.

6. **Associate yourself with good memories (SAVOURING).** Generally, people get negative thoughts while alone, especially when they are not doing any work. Associating oneself with positive memories can be done in several ways. That's why Indic scholars have valued self-study (swadhyaya) and the company of the holy (satsang) as elements of positive living.

7. **Capitalize on positive emotions.** Dealing with negative emotion is a formidable challenge. Research has shown that *five* positive comments can neutralize the adverse impact of *one* negative comment. Hence it is better to spread more and more positive emotions. In this context, the role of smile is significant. Generally, people think that we smile when we are happy. Though this is true, it is equally true that we are happy when we smile. It is not that mood always brings positive physical gesture; positive physical gesture can also induce positive mood. Hence keep smiling always.

■

Performance Excellence

The defining slogan in the modern workplace is more, bigger, faster. There are more customers to please, more e-mails to answer, more phone calls to return, more tasks to do, more meetings to attend, and more places to visit. The technologies that make instant communication possible anywhere, at any time, speed up decision making, create efficiencies, and fuel a global market place. But too much of a thing may become a bad thing. Left unmanaged and unregulated, these same technologies have the potential to overwhelm us. The relentless urgency that characterizes most corporate cultures undermines creativity, quality, engagement, thoughtful deliberation, productivity, and ultimately, performance.

The consulting firm Towers Perrin's most recent global workplace study bears this out. Conducted in 2007-2008, before the worldwide recession, it looked at some 90,000 employees in eighteen countries. Only 20 percent of them felt fully engaged, 40 percent were enrolled, and 38 percent were disengaged. More than a hundred studies have demonstrated similar gloomy picture of the modern era.

The Ericsson Study

In 1993, Anders Ericsson, a leading researcher in expert performance and a professor in Florida State

University, conducted an extraordinary study designed to explore the power of practice among violinists. Ericsson divided thirty young violinists at the Music Academy of Berlin into three separate groups, based on ratings from their professors.

The "best" group consisted of those destined to eventually become professional soloists. The "good" violinists were those expected to have careers playing as part of orchestras. The third group, recruited from the academy, was headed for careers as music teachers. All three groups had begun playing violin around the age of eight.

Vast amount of data was collected on each of the participants. All participants kept diary of their activities, hour by hour, over the course of an entire week. They were also asked to rate each hour's primary activity on three measures using a scale of 1 to 10. The first one was how important the activity was to improve their performance on the violin. The second was how difficult they found it to do. The third was how intrinsically enjoyable they found the activity.

The top two groups, both destined for professional careers, turned out to practice an average of twenty-four hours a week. The future music teachers, by contrast, put in just over nine hours, or about a third of the amount of time as the top two groups. This difference was undeniably dramatic and does suggest how much practice matters. But equally fascinating was the relationship Ericsson found between practice and intermittent rest.

All of the thirty violinists agreed that "practice alone" had the biggest impact on improving their performance as violinists. On an average, those on the top two groups slept 8 – 6 hours a day – nearly an hour longer than those in the music teacher group. The top two groups also took considerably more daytime naps than did the lower-rated group.

Great performance, Ericsson Study suggests, work more intensely than most of us do but also recover more deeply. The best violinists figured out, intuitively, that they generated the highest return on their investment by working intensely, without interruption, for no more than ninety minutes at a time and no more than 4 hours a day. They also recognized it was essential to take time, intermittently, to rest and refuel.

It is important to recognize that doing an activity for a long time is no guarantee that one will do it well.

We are not meant to rest solely at night. Basic rest activity cycle implies the ninety-minute period during which we move through the five stages of sleep. It is suggested that we experience a parallel ninety-minute cycle in our working life. At night, we move from light to deep sleep. During the day, we oscillate every ninety minutes or so from higher to lower alertness. We call these "ultradian" cycle, which literally means "less than a day".

■

The Second Brain in the Gut

A decade ago, the idea that the bacteria in our gut could influence our behaviour and mental health was seen as very vague. Today, it is well-established that the trillions of microbes in the gastrointestinal tract – collectively known as the **microbiome** influence health in countless ways. Inside the gut, those microscopic organisms program the developing immune system, help us make nutrients, defend against infection and produce neurochemicals important for brain function.

In the past several years, researchers have compiled convincing evidence that suggest the gut and its resident microorganisms influence mental health and cognition as well. Specialists refer to this as the microbiome-gut-brain axis, and that axis is bidirectional. The microbiome and gut are communicating with the brain, and conversely the brain is communicating with the gut and the microbiome. But when it comes to understand how those players communicate, researchers have a lot to sort out.

Research has already uncovered digestive and immune benefits of probiotics, live microorganisms in food and supplements that benefit the health of their hosts. As scientists learn more about the gut-brain connection, they are moving closer to the prospect of treating psychiatric and behavioural disorders with "dietary changes" or "**psychobiotics**" supplements filled with brain-benefitting microbes.

Gut-Brain Connection

For many decades, scientist have observed links between the gut and the nervous system. Researchers have described an important **second brain** in the gut, a complex network of neurons and neurotransmitters known as the entric nervous system. Meanwhile, scientists have noted that gut problems and mental health disorders often coincide. There are a number of different kinds of evidence for this gut-brain connection.

People with gastrointestinal disorders have higher-than-average rate of neuropsychiatric problems such as bipolar depression, while people with schizophrenia often have blood markers suggestive of gastrointestinal inflammation. People with autism spectrum disorders have higher states of gastro intestinal problems than the general population.

Researchers have identified a suite of potential mechanism to explain these patterns. Messages travel from the digestive tract in the brain along the vagus nerve, which forms a direct highway from gut to brainstem. There is also evidence that bacteria in the gut can generate metabolites that can circulate through the blood into the brain. Inflammation is another possible connection, as immune-signaling molecules and even immune cells can move from the other parts of the body into the brain and affect neural functions. It seems that there are many mechanisms, but we need more clarity on how they actually work.

Lowerp and his colleagues have studied whether beneficial bacteria can help reduce stress-related pathology in mice. They used an established model for triggering psychological stress by housing the mice to colonies with a dominant aggressive mouse. Normally, subordinate mice in this condition show signs of anxiety and develop colitis, an inflammation of the colon. The researchers injected some beneficial bacteria into stressed mice. The treated mice showed less anxiety and fear.

Therapeutic Potential

Other researchers are also beginning to explore the microbiome-gut-brain axis in humans. One study examined the effects of the gut bacteria. The researchers found that the probiotics improved the outcomes by modulating immune system. Other psychologists are trying to identify psychobiotics that would produce mental health benefits.

While much of the research thus far has identified how changes in the microbiome might affect the brain, other researchers are looking at the question in reverse. Can changing behaviour alter the microbiome and improve gut health?

Mayer and his colleagues at the University of Buffalo, finished a study of cognitive-behavioural therapy (CBT) aimed at reducing gastrointestinal problems and increasing coping skills. They found that microbiome could predict who would respond best to CBT. Among those respondents, the intervention actually altered the composition of their microbiome. This suggests a top-down effect.

If we change autonomous nervous activity by decreasing anxiety and increasing coping skills, the signals get from the brain down to the microbiome in the gut. It is not just the microbes talking to the brain. The brain has a big part in the conversation as well.

Experts still need to sort out where that conversation

begins. Are their brain changes first that signal to the gut and the microbes and alter their behaviour? Or the change are in the gut first? It seems that the model is circular, so we can't say which is the chicken and which is the egg.

Take Aways

Most likely, there are several healthy microbiomes. Perhaps western microbiome is typically much less than those of agrarian societies. This could be due to Westerners' higher consumption of high-fat, low fiber foods, as well as their use of antibiotics.

Doctors that treat diabetes or heart disease have already come around to understanding that diet is an important factor. The tried-and true advice of a high-fiber, low-sugar, mostly plant-based diet can benefit patients body and mind. Diet alone isn't going to cure mental illness, but it can make other therapies work better.

This is a fast-moving world. It is likely that psychologists would extend their help to a new field by designing and developing psychobiotics – healthy microbiome in the future.

Genes Are Not Destiny

It is a folk-belief that children come into the world with preexisting temperaments and emotional styles. It is believed that temperaments and emotional styles are shaped by the genes children inherit from their parents. Since infants and children have vey limited life-experiences, this belief is strengthened. Furthermore, studies comparing identical twins with fraternal twins provide some evidence that genes push us to be happy or unhappy, shy or bold, anxious or mellows. These studies argue that identical twins arise from a single fertilized egg and thus have identical gene sequence – those ribbons of chemical "letters" designated A, T, C and G that spell out what the gene does (what protein the gene codes for). Fraternal twins come from two different eggs fertilized by two different sperm and thus have the same degree of genetic relatedness as non-twin sibling, sharing roughly half the genes that come in different forms.

Many human genes come in only as a single variety, so no matter how two people are related, they have identical copies of such genes. Identical twins are thus, twice as similar genetically as non-twin siblings and should, thus, be about twice as similar as fraternal twins that have a genetic component.

Twin studies have been considered as a primary

source of genetic inference. Among the traits that are more similar in identical twins than in fraternal twins, and thus have a strong genetic basis, are shyness, sociability, emotionality, tendency to experience distress, adaptability, impulsivity, and the balance between positive and negative emotions.

The genetic contribution varies from 20 percent to 60 percent (about one-fifth to three-fifth). Whether this seems to high or low depends on the perspective. A strong genetic determinist would regard anything below 100 percent as very low, while an environmentalist would see even 20 percent as very high. To define the boundaries, the heritability of sickle-cell disease is 100 percent, while the heritability of a specific religious belief is close to zero.

Although many people view that every trait is a product of our inherited DNA, this is not so. *Genes are not our masters*. For example, schizophrenia has a strong genetic component. But one identical twin has the fifty-fifty chance of developing the disease. Depression has a modest genetic component. Yet it seems to vary by sex. In women the heritability of depression is about 40 percent, while in men it is about 30 percent. Genetic propensities can aim a child down a path that leads to a particular emotional style, but certain experiences and environment can move the child off that path.

Study of the Innate Basis

The pioneering study of the innate basis was undertaken by Jerry Kagan of Harvard University. Kagan was very passionate about his research on how a child's temperament develops. He pioneered the study of *behavioural inhibition*, a form of anxiety. The term describes the propensity to freeze in response to something novel or unfamiliar. In everyday terms, it looks a lot like *shyness*. Kagan was the first scientist to systematically examine the behavioural and biological correlates of individual difference among young children with respect to shyness.

Kagan assessed shyness when children were very young and again when in their early twenties. Kagan had parents describe their children and pre-adults. He himself observed them and obtained fMRI of their brains. The latter showed that young adults who were categorized as strongly inhibited as toddlers showed heightened activation of the amygdala compared with those who were uninhibited as toddlers. The amygdala plays a key role in fear and anxiety, responding to threatening events in the environment. Heightened activation in the amygdala reflects an important characteristic of behaviourally inhibited children and adults. The bottom line of Kagan's work: Behavioural inhibition is a stable feature of temperament. The shy five-year-old becomes the shy fifteen-year-old; the shy fifteen-year-old becomes the shy twenty-year-old. Kagan's work during the 1980s and 1990's became a part of the popular culture: *Born shy, always shy*.

But then a revolution swept through genetics, and the dogma that "genetic equals unchangeable" was toppled. Scientists made two startling and related discoveries that a *genetic trait will be expressed or not depending on the environment in which a child grows up and that the actual gene – the double helix that winds through every single one of our cells – can be turned on or off depending on the experiences we have.*

Contrary to the popular belief that we are stuck with the genetically given traits, for life, even genetically based traits can be dramatically modified by how parents, teachers and caregivers treat children and by the experiences children have.

Nurture Versus Nature

The reason genetically based traits can be altered is that the mere presence of a gene is not a sufficient condition for the trait for which it codes to be expressed. A gene must also be turned on and studies of both people and lab animals have shown that life experiences can turn genes on or off.

That became clear from studies of a gene that became notorious in the late 1980's when scientists began studying an extended Dutch family that included fourteen men who had committed impulsive, aggressive crimes. In 1998, scientists reported that all fourteen had the identical form of a gene on the X chromosome. The gene makes an enzyme called MAOA or monoamine oxidase A, an enzyme that metabolizes neurotransmitters such as serotonin, norepinephrine, and dopamine. The normal or long version of the gene produce lots of MAOA, the aberrant, or short form produces low amounts. The more MAOA enzyme in the brain, the faster these neurotransmitters are broken down.

About one-third of people have the short form of the MAOA gene, while two-thirds have the long form. Studies in animals had linked low MAOA levels, typical of the short form of the gene, to aggression. When MAOA is in short supply the brain remains jacked up on neurochemical in a way that induces aggression. Indeed, men with the short form of the MAOA gene tend to have a hair-trigger response to threat, as measured by a surge in activity in the brain's fear region (amygdala) at the sight of an angry face. This explains the violence committed by that Dutch family. The MAOA gene became known as the "Violence gene".

But then came a remarkable study. Scientists determined the MAOA status – benign long form or notorious short form of the gene – of 442 males in New Zealand. The scientist collected criminal and other public records to determine which of them had exhibited antisocial and criminal behaviours by age twenty-six. Scientists also conducted psychological assessment to ascertain whether each had antisocial personality disorder or adolescent conduct disorder. They interviewed at least one person who knew him well. Sixty-three percent of men had the high-activity form of the MAOA gene; 37 percent had the low-activity form. Here was the surprise. There was no statistically significant association between MAOA gene and status and antisocial behaviour. That is, sometimes low-activity – MAOA boys grew up to be criminals or delinquents, and sometimes they did not. But the "sometimes" was eye-opening. If a man with the low-activity MAOA gene has been abused as a child, as 8 percent had been, he was extremely likely to exhibit antisocial behaviour. Those with the exact same gene who had been loved and cared for, which described 64 percent of the men in the study, had no greater risk of antisocial behaviour than high-activity MAOA males. Genes alone did not increase the risk of delinquency and criminality that required a bad environment too.

The scientists followed up this study by looking at the same New Zealanders to see whether a similar nurture-nature dance was going on with another gene that had been linked to behaviour, namely, the serotonin transporter gene. This gene, located on chromosome 17, makes an enzyme that whisks serotonin, out of synapse. It thus has essentially the opposite effect of the popular antidepressants called SSRIs (Selective Serotonin Reuptake Inhibitors), which keeps serotonin in synapse longer. Not surprisingly, a short version of the gene, which results in less serotonin transporter being produced, has been linked to depression. But again, the scientists showed that **genes are not destiny.** Of men with the short version of the transporter gene, only those who had suffered, stressful life events in their early twenties had a high risk of depression. Having the "depression gene" without stressful events meant no risk of depression.

These were the first hints that our emotional and psychological fate does not lie solely with the twists of the double helix. Depending on the experience a child has had, the genetic basis for shyness or aggression or delinquency might or might not manifest. Whether you store your music on an ipod or a CD, what music we hear depends on what music gets played. **Genes load the gun, but only the environment can pull the trigger.**

Predictor of Gene Expression

How does the life we lead turn the genes off or leave them on? Back in the 1990s, biologist **Michael Meany** provided some satisfactory answer. Meany was studying rats. Some rats were extremely anxious and aggressive, while others were non-anxious and mellow. The anxious rats were highly inhibited and neurotic; they released a flood of stress hormones called glucocorticoids, which get the heart pumping. The other rats were relaxed, they explored as happily as teenage girls in a new shopping mall. When given an electric shock, they released only a small amount of glucocorticoid stress hormone.

In the mid 1990s, Meany discovered that the reason some rats had tolerated stress is that they produce fewer glucocorticoids in response to stress. A little bit of stress hormone goes a long way, so less of it floods their bodies in response to a stressful experience. With less stress hormone coursing through their blood, the rats seem more mellow, more jumpy, less fearful, less neurotic. In contrast, some rats are more sensitive to stress hormones is that their brains contain more receptors for them, in the hippocampus. Receptors, as their names imply serve as docking stations for glucocorticoids. With profusion of receptors, the body does not need to produce as much stress hormone to get the message across.

Meany discovered the reason some rats had more glucocorticoid receptors in their brains, and hence tolerated stress better, was that their mothers lavished licks and grooming on them. This experience made a lifelong difference in the baby rats, programming their brains to shrug off stressful experience. Pups whose mothers had licked and groomed them grew up to be competent. But baby rats whose mothers rarely licked and groomed them grew up to be fearful and stressed out.

Meany made another bold attempt to look into the issue of nurture's effect on nature. Generally neurotic anxious female rats gave birth to neurotic babies; nonneurotic mothers gave birth to nonneurotic babies. Meany opened a sort of rodent adoption agency,having neurotic mothers raise pups born to mellow mothers and mellow mothers raise pups born to neurotic ones. Nurture trumped nature. Pups born to anxious, neurotic, neglectful mothers but raised by attentive mothers grew up to be laid-back and well-adjusted babies. They were as happy as their adoptive mothers. Pups born to nurturing mellow mothers but raised by neglectful mothers grew up as neurotic babies. *The rats had inherited a behaviour – from mothers whose genes they did not share.* **It was a triumph of nurture over nature.**

■

Adding Life to Years

The study of the positive aspects of aging is only several decades old. It will become a primary focus of psychological science in near future. The life expectancy is showing upward trend almost everywhere in this world. The expressions such as *old age,* gerontology, *geriatric care* and so on are gradually becoming obsolete. There are replaced by positive terms such as *positive aging, healthy aging,* and *successful aging*. Psychologists prefer to use the late adulthood in the place of old age.

The basic objective of this article is to highlight certain lifestyle guidelines that are intended for "adding life to years". Although there has been a systematic attempt to understand both the process of old age depression and successful aging, the purpose is not to describe the studies and their findings. Rather the goal is to generate guidelines for navigating our life course in a difficult world.

While the present focus is placed on the positivity, a brief note on the darker side of the life is needed to highlight the positive.

The Depressive Cycle

Depression is comparable to cough and cold experienced in our day-to-day lives. It does not matter if birds of depression fly over our heads. Yet we must not allow them to build their nests in our heads. Everyone experiences depression occasionally, though some people have a greater share of it. It is a common belief that elderly people experience it more often. It may be due to physical infirmity and illness, loneliness, loss of friends and relatives, and other uncontrollable factors.

It is basically a mood disorder. It may take three different forms. It is greater in women than in men. The first form is a hypo variety characterized by withdrawal and low social contact. The second form is hyper variety called mania. Maniacs show irritability, talk a lot and behave in an aggressive manner. Many depressives show bipolar symptoms, they show severe mood swings from low activity to hyper activity.

Although many elderly depressives report memory loss, that may not be true. Lab studies do not reveal significant difference between depressive elderly and nondepressive elderly. Their perception may be the result of their low confidence. Similarly, they pretend as if they have not listened, even if they have listened. This is because of their lowered activity and lack of confidence.

The remediation attempts have been made from several quarters. Medicines have been used, yet it is not without complication. It may lead to the problem of dependability. Chronic use may lead to respiratory problems.

Psychologists recommend behavioural medicine. Situations or factors associated with depression are to be identified first. Then appropriate steps can be taken to remove or to reduce the intensity of those factors. If loneliness is the root, provide social contact, talk to him/her, provide work/job that is interesting to the person.

The present author believes that adaptive explanatory styles are important to combat depression. If bad (negative) events happen, individuals ought to explain the event in terms of external (other people are responsible), unstable (the event is temporary) and specific (the event would adversely affect only one aspect of my life) factors. If good (positive) events happen, adaptive styles would involve internal (I have a role in getting it done), stable (the effect is relatively permanent) and global (it would influence many aspects of life). In sum, depressive individuals need to be trained to explain negative events in terms of external, unstable and specific parameters whereas they need to explain positive events in terms of internal (personal), stable (permanent), and global (pervasive) factors.

Since the present consideration is refocused on positive parameters of later adulthood, a number of salient features of this New Look Approach are indicated.

Positive Aging

There are two bench-marking studies in the international context. As indicated earlier, the objectives of these studies are geared to identifying components of successful aging.

The MacArthur Foundation Study. The MacArthur Foundation undertook a mega-study spanning from 1988 to 1996. They selected 1,189 healthy adult volunteers (aged 70 to 79 years) from a sample of 4,030 adults. Each participant was interviewed for about 90 minutes in the beginning, subsequently brief interviews were conducted within the project period of seven years.

The study identified *three* components of positive aging:
- Avoiding disease
- Engagement with life
- Maintaining high cognitive and physical function

The findings can schematically be presented in the following Exhibit:

Components of Positive Aging		
1. Avoiding disease		
2. Engagement with life	Social support	Socioemotional Instrumental
	Productivity Creativity)	
3. High levels of cognitive & physico functionary		

The components identified are comparative to abilities, health and well-being. Life engagement is a form of love, work and play. Life engagement has two components: social support and productivity (creativity). Social support is manifested in two forms: First, it denotes socioemotional support (liking and loving). It is desirable that amount of love given should be proportional to the amount of love received. The second form of social support refers to the instrumental social support. It is the amount of assistance received when needed.

An interesting finding in MacArthur Foundation study was the gender's role. It was shown that men received emotional support primarily from their spouses. Women drew more heavily on their friends and relatives and children for their emotional support.

Sustained physical activity (an aspect of productive activity) helps to maintain healthy functioning.

The Harvard Study. Another landmarking study in the context of positive aging is known as Harvard's Adult Development Study. A renowned psychologist George Vaillant pioneered this study. Initially Deans of various

schools of Harvard identified healthy adults who were likely to make successful transitions to their seventies and eighties. This empirical study identified *lifestyle predictors* of healthy aging. The list includes:
- Not smoking or stopping smoking while young
- Coping well (with mature defenses)
- Not abusing alcohol
- Maintaining a healthy weight
- Stable marriage
- Exercise

As an additional point to this study, Vaillant (2002) greatly emphasize the role of *altruism* (helping without any expectation of reciprocation) and humour.

Concluding Remark

In addition to the findings of MacArthur and Harvard study, the importance of experiencing positive emotions is to be underlined. In a magnificent study, Danner and his associates studied autobiographies of 180 catholic nuns. When nuns enter into church life, each of them submits a 2-page write-up indicating their intention and interest. With the permission of the church administration, researchers obtained those write-ups from the archive and analyzed them.

More specifically, the researchers looked into the extent of use of positive adjectives in their write-ups. It was clearly shown that the extent of positive adjectives was a stable predictor of their longevity and happiness. However, it is important to note that it is not the intensity of positive affect that counts; rather the frequency of moderate positive emotion is a surer determinant of health and happiness in later years.

Despite the recommendations, many people may

wonder about the mechanism of controlling the negative. For them, a closer look at the statement of Vaillant (2002) is a constant reminder:

Statement of a renowned researcher of successful aging (VAILLANT, 2002)

"Constrain to all expectations, I seem to grow happier as I grow older. I think that the world has been sold on the theory that youth is marvelous but old age is terror. On the contrary, it has taken me 60 years to learn how to live reasonably well, to do my work and cope with my inadequacies.

For me, youth was a woeful time-sick parents, war, relative poverty, the miseries of learning a profession, a mistake of a marriage, self-doubts, and blundering around. Old age is knowing what I am doing, the respect of others, a relatively sane financial base, a loving wife, and the realization that what I can't beat. I can endure.

George Vaillant

Awareness of Death

People hold different attitudes towards death. Ravi is in his late thirties and he shivers at the mention of the word *death*. Those who know him well say this reaction may have something to do with the tragic death of his elder brother in a car accident when Ravi was a young boy. Ravi refuses to attend funerals, even for his close friends. One can only speculate how Ravi would react if his wife or children should die before he does.

Mita, a widow in her late seventies, maintains a very different attitude towards death. She is grieving over the recent loss of her husband, to whom she was happily married for 50 years. She talks openly with her friends about how much she misses him. She regularly offers flowers at the photo. Knowing that her husband never liked her being alone, she periodically visits friends and relatives. She sometimes talks to herself: "Don't worry, I will be with you one day".

Which of these two attitudes would you endorse? Death is a difficult concept to define. A common *definition* of death is the cessation of life as measured by the absence of breathing, heartbeat, and electrical activity of the brain. Some of us would prefer to think in line with Ravi while others would endorse Mita's style. Perhaps most of us fall somewhere in between these two extremes.

Actually, some denial of death, such as in Ravi, is necessary and normal to function effectively. Death, especially the possibility of our own death, is such a harsh reality that few people would face it directly. Denial helps to keep our anxiety level at a low, manageable level. Denial also helps to avoid thoughts of being separated from loved ones, whose relationship is so vital for our self-esteem and well-being. There is another reason for not thinking about death; it is futile to think about the inevitable. In this world, nothing is certain except death.

An excessive or inappropriate denial has a cost factor. It increases vulnerability. People who consistently reassure themselves that it would not happen to them untimely may become careless. They may continue to smoke and drink; they may eat junk foods. They may get into health risks. They may also postpone doing something meaningful.

Despite attempts at denial, each of us has some awareness of our own mortality. For instance, suppose you are asked, "How often do you think about your own death?" If your reply is "once in a while", a lot of people belong to your group. About half of the people asked this question answer "occasionally". Another fourth say "frequently" or "very frequently" whereas another fourth claim they rarely have thoughts about their own death.

Actually, our personal awareness of death fluctuates somewhat everyday. Most of the time, we have very little awareness of death. We avoid thinking about the possibility of our death and deny that someday our lives must end. The more intense the denial, the lower is our awareness of death. Other days, we are more aware that our life span is limited. Perhaps we have just seen a gory automobile accident, or someone we know has discovered he or she has a serious illness. When people are questioned directly about death, they rarely admit being fearful of it. But indirect methods reveal that they are fearful.

The personal awareness of death also varies somewhat by age. Interestingly, people in their late twenties are the most fearful of all, perhaps partly because they have most of their lives ahead of them. The natural calamities like floods, cyclones, earthquakes and hurricanes and other catastrophic events such as terrorist attack trigger death-awareness. As individuals reach late adulthood, they generally think about death more often and talk about it more openly. The increase in chronic illness and the death of close friends at this age are all reminders that death is the natural end of life. Finally, older people are usually less fearful of death than other age groups. After all, they have already lived a reasonably long life and may have less to look forward to. Also, those with a deep religious faith, including belief in some kind of afterlife, are generally less fearful of death. Such a belief may provide an important mechanism for dealing with the anxieties of aging and death.

Near Death Experience

Suppose somebody meets an automobile accident, looses consciousness and is taken to hospital critically injured, the individual is put on a life-support system that keeps him/her alive. After a couple of days, the individual regains consciousness, only to discover that he/she almost died. There is a good chance that he/she would have had a **near-death experience** – the distinctive state of recall associated with being brought back to life from the verge of death.

Accounts of these experiences show striking similarities. Initially, individuals experience a detachment from their bodies. There may be a lot of variation in what they report. Many people may brand their reports as illusions and delusions. Yet they exhibit some tangible transformations after they go through near-death experience.

For most people, the near-death experience brings a profound change in attitudes. They not only become less fearful of death but are also more concerned with loving and valuing the life they have. There is also an increase in spirituality. They show more concerns for others and less concerns for material.

No matter what their age, race, sex, or education level is, the experience seems transforming. Alcoholics find themselves unable to like beer, hardened criminals opt for a life of helping others. Atheists embrace religion or talk about spiritual matters. Although people having near-death experiences report a number of unbelievable spiritual encounters, modern psychologists are attempting to explain the changes in terms of neurological modifications in the brain.

The Stages of Experience of Dying

The sequence of physiological and psychological changes experienced by individuals who are dying is interesting.

One of the best-known pioneers in this field is Elizabeth Kubler-Ross. She and her associates interviewed more than 500 terminally ill patients at the University of Chicago hospital. She found that even if people are not told of the seriousness of their illness, they usually guess the approximate time of their death. Compared to the past tradition, doctors today are more likely to reveal to a patient his or her terminal prognosis. Hence, there is a growing realization that when persons indicate a willingness to know the truth about their impending death, it may be wiser to give the relevant information than to protect them with a conspiracy of concealment. This also provides them with some time to get their affairs in order, for example, write a will if they do not have one.

Kubler-Ross noted that individuals tend to go through several stages in dying, although there is considerable overlap between these stages. The first stage consists of a **denial of death** with people characteristically feeling: *"No, not me; this cannot happen to me"*. Such denial protects them from deep emotions associated with death. It provides time to cope with the disturbing facts. Later, individuals tend to show small signs that they are now willing to talk about death. Yet at this stage friends and professionals should talk about it and for a few minutes at a time allowing the dying to make the needed adjustment.

In the second stage, denial eventually gives way to the emotion of anger and **resentment**, *especially towards individuals who are healthy*. The sight of others enjoying their health evokes envy, jealousy and anger. The dying often take their feelings out on those closest to them, mostly because of what these people represent – life and health. Consequently, it is important for those nearby not to take these remarks personally, but to help the dying persons express their feelings.

The third stage consists of attempts to **bargain for time** in which the dying individuals *attempt to negotiate with others* (e.g., O 'God' help me to live. If I live longer, I would not waste time. I would devote time for the welfare of others). When individuals tend to drop the "but" and admit, "Yes, I am dying", they enter the fourth stage" **depression**. *It is characterized by intense and sometimes unrealistic sadness*. In a sense, this is a natural response to the threat of losing one's life. It is very important to allow the dying person to grieve and express sadness. It is necessary for family and friends as well as professionals to learn to accept their own feeling about death so that they can help dying people accept their own impending death without dwelling on it unduly.

The final stage is the **acceptance of death**, though not all dying persons reach this stage. By this time, *most people who are dying have pretty much accepted death and are disengaged from others*. They ask only for fewer visitors. In fact much of the pain of dying comes from mental anguish, especially the fear of being separated from loved ones.

However, the experience of dying is not a fixed, inevitable process and many people do not follow these stages. For some, anger remains the dominant mood throughout, whereas others are depressed until the end. Individual differences are more pronounced across age, sex, personality and cultural identities.

What is your level of death anxiety?
Instruction: For each of the following statements, indicate your degree of agreement / disagreement according to the following norm.
Indicate '1' if you strongly disagree.
Indicate '2' if you disagree.
Indicate '3' if you slightly disagree
Indicate '4' if you cannot decide.
Indicate '5' if you slightly agree.
Indicate '6' if you agree.
Indicate '7' if you strongly agree.

Statements
- I feel uncomfortable while reading materials on death and dying.
- I am distressed by the thought of planning my own funeral.
- When I know someone is terminally ill, I find it difficult to visit.
- It is difficult for me to discuss the arrangements to be made after my death.
- I prefer not to attend funerals or other death-related events.
- Thoughts of my own death trouble me.
- I hesitate to venture out for adventures.
- The sight of funerals bothers me.
- I am disturbed by the thought that nothingness follows death.
- I experience death-related anxiety.

Interpretation
Sum your ratings (1 through 7) across all 10 statements and interpret in terms of the following key:
70-55= You have high levels of death anxiety.
54-40= You have moderate levels of death anxiety.
39-25= You are neither comfortable or uncomfortable.
24-10= You are not particularly distressed by the topic of death.

Value Education

Education is a process of transformation. Although a large number of definitions of education can be cited, two definitions stand out. George Bernard Shaw defined education in an interesting manner: "Education is that what remains after you forget all that has been taught in schools and colleges". Our Indic scholars defined education as a liberating force (*sa vidya ya bimuktaye*). In essence, both the definitions underline the core elements of residual effect. Education is neither the ability to solve mathematical problems nor the ability to memorize poems. It is a movement towards human values and virtues. It denotes the sublimation of emotion. It represents the improvisation of cognitive, affective and psychomotor capacities inherent in human beings.

The Components of Positive Educational Environment

The quality of students depends on the positive attributes of educational environment. Every biological organism develops within the context of ecological systems that support or stifle its growth. Just as we need to understand the ecology of the ocean or the forest if we wish to understand the development of a fish or a tree, we need to understand the ecology of educational environment if we want to understand how students develop.

Urie Bronfenbrenner's influential *bioecological theory* describes the range of interacting influences that affect a developing person. According to Bronfenbrenner, development occurs through increasingly complex processes of interaction between a developing person and the immediate every-day environment- processes that are affected by more remote contexts of which the person is not aware. He identifies five interlocking contextual systems, from the most intimate to the broadest – the *microsystem, mesosystem, exosystem, macrosystem,* and *chronosystem.*

A *microsystem* is a pattern of activities, roles and relationships within a system (such as home and educational system) in which a human being functions on a first-hand, day-to-day basis. It is through the microsystem that more distant influences, such as social institutions and cultural values, reach the developing individual. A *mesosystem* is the linkage between two or more microsystems that contain the individual. An exosystem is also the linkage between two or more setting, but one of the settings does not contain the person. For examples, colleagues of parents or teachers of students may try to influence students by their observations and comments. The macrosystem entails broader socio-cultural environment which influences learners. Finally, the chronosystem defines the spirit of time. Although these settings influence the growth of learners, the role of family and educational institution is a primary consideration.

It is a common observation that the basic aim of education is the enhancement of students' strength rather than the remediation of weaknesses. For this, a foundation of care, trust and respect for diversity is needed. However, this kind of positive class-room ambience is possible only when morality and ethics in education is preserved and promoted.

Morality and Ethics

Needless to say that man stands out distinct from other living species on account of the characteristic possessions namely: ability to reason and judge an action or a state of affairs as good or bad, desirable or undesirable, beautiful or ugly. Rationality discloses 'man' as a thinking being whereas the latter introduces man as a valuing-animal despite differences in details about what is considered as right or wrong, beautiful or ugly by individuals. *The very capacity to make such valuations* is universal. The act of 'reasoning' and 'valuing' disclose second-order consciousness. That is why logic, morality and ethics remain as integral parts of human behaviour.

The highest end of reason is to arrive at truth. The supreme end of the valuing faculty is to realize what is ultimately 'good' and that of aesthetic faculty is to discover the beautiful. Thus Truth, Beauty and Goodness are intrinsically valuable. Thought, speech and action are said to have values only when they help one achieve the highest values.

Man is essentially a moral being. Non-humans sometimes cannot transcend the first-order of the consciousness. They are activated by instincts and antecedent events. The notions of 'ought' and 'ought-not' has a great deal of application for humans. Ethics as a study examines the very nature and dynamics of moral valuation.

Ethics

Ethics involves critical thinking about human action;

it is a step removed from the domain of action. It examines the nature of moral judgment. Different norms are implicitly or explicitly invoked in ethical consideration. It addresses such fundamental questions as what is the nature of ethical norms? Are norms ontologically neutral? Are values relative or absolute? Is the distinction between good and evil fundamental? Can there be an objective ground of morality? What are the presuppositions of moral discourse?

Both the discussion on morality and ethics bring home the necessity of morality and ethics in our individual and collective life. This is more so in our educational setting. It is greatly realized that educational objectives cannot be fulfilled without moral and ethical values in educational sphere in general and class-room behavior in particular.

The study of human values was a core concern of philosophers. There are many discursive models of human values suggested by philosophers. Broadly speaking, philosophers have equated education with philosophy: they have viewed that the purpose of education is to stimulate the natural goodness in man. Sociologists, on the contrary, have viewed men as inherently wicked. According to sociological approach, the purpose of education is to foster socialization which correct individuals. However, behavioral scientists in general and psychologists in particular have started investigating the issue lately. There are a number of reasons for this late entry into an area which appears to be a complex domain.

Table – 1 Approaches to Value Education

Approach	Basic Assumption	Means Emphasized
Philosophical	Individual is innately good; The goodness has to be realized	Self-training and education which is synonymous with philosophy
Sociological	Individual is innately bad; Society corrects individuals through socialization	Right kind of socialization process; Right kind of roles by socializing agents such as family, institution etc.
Psychological		
Cognitive-Development	Natural and orderly unfolding of the conception of right and wrong	Enriched exposure
Social Learning	Learning through models, Observations, Examples	Appropriate role models

Behavioural scientists and psychologists tend to move from a conceptual level to an empirical level. Consequently they have attempted to define human values at an operational level and identify the correlates of human values. A fundamental question that has concerned psychologists involves the very basis of human values. Although knowledge and information in this area is far from being complete, a number of approaches have suggested the psychological basis of human values. Four fundamental approaches can be discussed.

Evolutionary Approach: Behavioural scientists in the past gave emphasis on the trait of aggressiveness as a fundamental attribute of human beings. It was argued that aggressiveness is helpful for adaptation and natural selection. Under the Darwinian influence, psychologists were led to believe that the trait of aggressiveness gets transmitted because of its adaptive value.

However, the works of sociobiologists have presented a different picture. More specifically, Wilson has carried out several laboratory experiments and has shown that altruism has a genetic basis. His work has persuaded researchers to look into the possibility of genetic transmission of several socially useful traits such as altruism.

The noted psychologist Campbell asserts that there is a balance between two parallel evolutions; the physical evolution and the moral evolution. According to Campbell, all human societies strive towards a balance between these two parallel evolutions.

Neuropsychological Approach: It can be argued that the utility of values and morality is likely to be represented at the neurophysiological level. The repetitive use of particular behavior gets represented at the neural level. Although representation of value-based behaviour has not been clearly evinced, but certain works in the area of emotional intelligence point to the possibility of value-based behaviour. Psychologists have argued that the human brain has functionally two minds: the thinking brain and the feeling brain. More importantly, the feeling brain evolved prior to the thinking brain. From this standpoint, feeling brain is older. Generally the right hemisphere of the brain and limbic system regulate human emotion.

Furthermore, a number of psychologists in recent years have shown that human success and adaptation is incomplete within the framework of rational intelligence. In other words, emotional intelligence is needed for better personal and collective life. Emotional intelligence involves a number of human values including tolerance, self-control and interpersonal sensitivity.

More recently, some neuropsychologist have spoken about spiritual intelligence. They have also identified a centre in the brain (a centre in the temporal lobe) that controls spiritual activities. It is shown that the centre of spiritual intelligence is well developed in case of persons with ethical spiritual background. However, further research is needed to draw definitive conclusions.

Developmental Approach: It is interesting to observe that children in all cultures go through some distinct stages of development as far as moral development is concerned. The eminent psychologist, Piaget, spoke about stage-wise development of children's cognitive growth. Kohlberg followed similar model and extended it to the case of moral development.

According to Kohlberg, there are three distinct phases of child's moral development (see the Tables). Each phase has two stages. Cross-cultural psychologists working with children have observed these phases such as preconventional, conventional and post-conventional. It is important to note that there is a sequence of these three phases in all cultures. The universality of this observation strengthens the significance of human values across cultures.

Table 2: Kohlberg's Theory of Moral Development

Level I Preconventional Morality	
Stage 1 Obedience and Punishment orientation	To avoid punishment, the child defers to prestigious or powerful people, usefully the parents. The morality of an act is defined by its physical consequences.
Stage 2 Naïve hedonistic and Instrumental orientation	The child conforms to gain rewards. The child understands reciprocity and sharing, but this reciprocity is manipulative and self-serving rather than based on a true sense of justice, generosity, sympathy, or compassion. It is a kind of bartering: I will lend you my bike if I can play with your wagon.
Level-II Conventional Morality: Conventional Rules and Conformity	
Stage 3 Good boy morality	The child's good behaviour is designed to maintain approval and good relations with others. Although the child is still basing judgments of right and wrong on other responses, he is concerned with their approval and disapproval rather than their physical power. It is to maintain goodwill that he conforms to families and friends' standards. However, the child is starting to accept others social regulations and to judge the goodness or badness of behaviour in terms of a person's intent to violate these rules.

Stage 4 Authority and morality that maintain the social order	The person blindly accepts social conventions and rules and believes that if society accepts these rules, they should be maintained to avoid censure. He now conforms not just to other individual's standards but to the social order. This is the epitome of 'law and order' morality, involving unquestioning acceptance of social regulations. The person judges behaviour as good according to whether it conforms to a rigid set of rules. According to Kohlberg, many people never go beyond this conventional level of morality.
Level-III Postconventional Morality: Self-Accepted Moral Principles	
Stage 5 Morality of contract, individual rights and democratically accepted law	People now have a flexibility of moral beliefs they lacked in earlier stages. Morality is based on an agreement among individuals to conform to norms that appear necessary to maintain the social order and the rights of others. However, because this is a social contract, it can be modified when people within a society rationally discuss alternatives that might be more advantageous to more members of the society.
Stage 6 Morality of individual principles and conscience	People conform both to social standards and to internalized ideals. Their intent is to avoid self-condemnation rather than criticism by others. People base their decisions on abstract principles involving justice, compassion, and equality. This is a morality based on respect for others. People who have attained this level of development will

Apart from the approaches relating to the significance of human values, some generalizations can be derived with respect to the value of education.

Techniques of Value Education

While human values are considered important, the learning of these values is not an automatic process. There are many barriers to the task of value education. However, a number of techniques based on psychological knowledge can be suggested.

Cognitive Technique: Values are some kind of constellation of several attitudes. We are aware that each attitude has three components; Cognitive (information), affect (feeling), and motivation (behaviour). Generally, these three components tend to exist in a state of balance. If imbalance is created, an attitude is changed so as to attain balance.

This technique can be used for inducing human

values. For example, a person has a negative information about values; he or she does not like it; he or she behaves in opposition to values. In this case, all the three components are in balance, but the balance can be disturbed when the person is given sufficient information about the importance of human values. This kind of exposure will create a state of imbalance. Consequently, it is likely that his or her feeling and motivation will change so that the balance is restored.

While using this technique, it is better to manipulate the affect (feeling) component. It has been shown that good literature, family drama and emotion provoking situation change a person's value system. The change agent needs to manipulate person's feeling to produce value-based behaviour.

Expectancy Technique: People are motivated towards activity which they consider important for the attainment of their important goals. It is a fact that different people have different priority system. A person does not use value-based behaviour until and unless he or she perceives its linkage with his or her important goals. For example, if a person feels that untruthfulness is instrumental to his or her achievement, the person will not use truthfulness. In other words, wrong connections have to be broken and new connections have to be strengthened to achieve success and happiness. Motivation would be stronger to follow these values.

Training Technique: it is possible to make use of purposive training programme to induce values. The effective method suggested by Indian thinkers and pursued by many people in different parts of India involves several mind-stilling exercises aimed at the inculcation of human values. In this method, there is no imposition from the outside. The individual spends time in meditation and self-reflection and a changed process automatically starts. The other methods are influence techniques. For instance, the change-agents in an organization may make use of several influence techniques. They may provide reward for value-based behaviour. They may also provide check points for correcting deviant behaviour. In sum, the creation of appropriate learning environment, the presence of role models and collaborative discussion are considered helpful in this context.

Table 3: Suggested Intervention Strategy Based on Psychological Principle

Levels of Operation	Target of Influence	Strategy	Outcomes
Individual Child	Cognition Feeling Behaviour	Active reading Value game Visuals	Changed behaviour
Parents	Cognition Feeling Behaviour	Group discussion	Improved awareness Behaviour change
Teachers	Cognition Feeling Behaviour	Group activity	Improved awareness Behaviour change
Community	Cognition Feeling Behaviour	Use of informal leaders	Improved awareness Behaviour change

Table 4: Pragmatic Approach

Direct Intervention	Indirect Intervention
(Value education as a part of Curriculum/ planned teaching activities)	Curriculum (Focusing on the value while teaching a curricular topic) Co-curriculum (Assigning value-oriented topics during co-curricular events such as debate and literary competitions) Incidental (Asking students to analyze certain incidents such as conflict between two groups of students)

In conclusion, it may be indicated that psychological research in the area of human values has a late entry. Although some of the fundamental questions have been answered, but many more have remained unanswered. It is expected that only the future research would clarify many issues surrounding the concept of human values.

Value Inclusion in Class-Room

Corrective socialization in the class-room setting is essential for value-inculcation. However, the successful implementation of this objective requires multi-strategy multi-level approach.

The philosophical approach advocates for self-purification methods for value-education. In the eight-fold path of yogic practice, *yama* and *niyam* constitute the initial steps. These are essentially external and internal disciplines. The sociological approach would stress the use of controls and disciplinary action for curbing negative behaviour. In contrast, psychological approach involves the change of cognitive restructuring and use of role models for value inclusion process.

However, it is important to recognize that the interventions aimed at inducing moral and ethical behaviours in students *only* would not generate satisfactory outcomes. Parents, teachers and relevant others must constitute the packaged target group for which value-education intervention is geared.

References :
- Emotional Intelligence – Deniel Goleman
- Psychology of Jean Piaget – Flavelt
- Moral Education – R. Sarangi
- Studies of Cross – Cultural Values – Schwdrtz

Avoiding Overthinking

Overthinking is thinking too much, needlessly, passively, endlessly, and excessively pondering its meanings, causes and consequences of your character, your feelings, and your problems: "Why am I so unhappy? What will happen to me if I lose my job? What did he really mean when he made that remark on me?"

Many of us believe that when we face a problem, we should think deeply to find a solution. Yes! But too much analysis is paralysis. Numerous studies over the past two decades have shown that overthinking ushers in a host of adverse consequences. It sustains and worsens sadness, fosters negatively biased thinking, impairs a person's ability to solve problems, saps motivation, and interferes with concentration and initiative. Moreover, although people have a strong sense that they are gaining insight into themselves and their problems during their ruminations, this is rarely the case. What they gain is a distorted, pessimistic perspective on their lives.

The combination of rumination and negative mood is toxic. Research shows that people ruminate while sad are likely to feel powerless, self-critical, pessimistic, and generally negatively biased. The evidence that overthinking is bad for you is not vast. If you are someone plagued by ruminations, you are unlikely to become happier before you can break that habit. If you are an overthinker, one of the secrets to your happiness is the ability to allay obsessive overthinking, to reinterpret and redirect your negative thoughts into more neutral or optimistic ones. Happy people have the capacity to direct and absorb themselves in activities that divert their energies and attention away from anxious ruminations.

Daily life is replete with minor upsets, hassles, and reversals. In most people's experiences, other unavoidable events include illness, rejection, failure, and sometimes devastating trauma. However, those who react strongly to life's ups and downs, who have got difficulty shaking off unavoidable information are unhappy people.

Becoming happier means learning how to disengage from overthinking about both major and minor negative experiences, learning to stop searching for all the leaks and cracks — at least for a time — and not let them affect how you feel about yourself and your life as a whole.

Shaking Off Ruminations

Ruminations can be very compelling. You may combat overthinking and ruminations by adopting some effective strategies. Some of the strategies are listed below.

Cut loose. First, you need to free yourself from the clutch of your rumination. The first strategy to arrest overthinking is simple: **distract, distract, distract.** The distracting activity you select must be engrossing enough so that you don't have the opportunity to lapse back into ruminations. Good bets are activities that make you feel happy, curious, peaceful, amused, or proud. Read or watch something that's funny, listen to a song that's transporting, meet a friend for tea, do a physical activity that gets your heart rise up. It doesn't matter what you do, as long as it absorbs you, compels you, and isn't potentially harmful.

Although distraction seems like almost too simple, short-term solution or quick-fix, the positive emotions that it begets can "debias" your thinking (opening up a new, more objective, and more positive perspective on your troubles) and hone resources and skills (like creativity, sociability and problem-solving skills) that would be useful in future. Even a transient lift in mood can make you feel energetic.

The second strategy is the **"Stop" technique**, in which you think, say, or even shout to yourself: "Stop" or "No". Use your intellectual power to think about something else — like your shopping list or what will you say when you call the man to repair your fridge. The technique is valuable in many situations, including moments when your thoughts wander even during a distracting pastime.

The third strategy directs us to set aside thirty minutes every day to do nothing but ruminating. Accordingly, if you find the negative thoughts pushing and pulling, you can truthfully tell yourself, "I can stop now, because I will have the opportunity to think about this later." Ideally, that thirty-minute period should be at a time of the day when you're not anxious or sad. More often than not, when the appointed time arrives, you will find it difficult and unnatural to force yourself to overthink.

The fourth strategy is to talk to a sympathetic and trusted person about your thoughts and problems. Choose carefully your sympathetic person. He or she must be able to think objectively, not make you feel even worse or end up ruminating out loud with you. You must not abuse this opportunity. If you bring your negative thoughts and worries ad infinitum, you may wear people out so much that they avoid you.

The final strategy involves writing. Whether in a handsome journal, in a computer file, or on a scrap of paper, writing out your ruminations can help you organize them, make sense of them, and observe pattern that you haven't perceived before. Writing is also a way to unburden yourself of your negative thoughts — to spill them on a page, so to speak — allowing you to move past them.

Problem-solving action. You need to gain a new perspective on yourself and on your life in general. Essentially you need to try to solve the very real, concrete problems that might inspire your overthinking. For example, even if you're feeling weighed down by your problems and responsibilities and are indecisive about what to do, take a small step now. Perhaps this entails making an appointment with a doctor (even if you are pessimistic about doctor's expertise). If you're hesitant, think of a person whom you highly respect and admire and ask yourself which solution he or she would choose. Don't wait for something to happen or someone else to step in and help you Act right away. Even small steps will improve your mood and self-regard.

Avoiding future overthinking. You need to learn how to avoid future overthinking trips. For example, write a list of situations (places, persons, and time) that appear to trigger your overthinking. If at all possible, avoid those situations. This is not different from what a smoker must do when quitting, avoiding locations, time of the day and specific people that set off his desire to smoke.

If you are determined, learn how to meditate. The skill involved in this relaxation technique can help you distance yourself from your worries and ruminations and impart a positive sense of well-being.

Take in the big picture. In addition to the strategies

discussed, one can combat overthinking with the help of a big picture. Will this matter in a year? Your answer will offer you a big picture view of your troubles and diminish your worries. If it remarkable how quickly things that seem so momentous and pressing this moment emerge as fairly trivial and insignificant. Sometimes when I am facing a horrendous week, I remind myself that I won't remember it one month, six months, or a year from now. (The more extreme version of this strategy is to use the deathbed criterion. Will it matter when you're on you deathbed?)

Another valuable approach is to distance yourself from rumination even further by contemplating your particular problem in the context of space and time. Visualize yourself (and the strains, worries, tribulations facing you) as a microscopic dot on earth, which is a tiny part of the Milky Way, which makes up an infinitesimal speck of the universe. This brings home the point that few things in life are so significant that they are worth overthinking.

Finally, if you resolve that the trouble you are enduring now is indeed significant and will matter in a year, then consider what experience it can teach you. Focusing on the lesson you can learn from a stress will help soften its blow. The lessons that these realities impart could be patience, perseverance, loyalty, or courage. Perhaps you are learning open-mindedness, forgiveness, generosity, or self-control.

■

Attitude of Gratitude

It is a truism that how you think — about yourself, your world, and other people — is more important to your well-being than the objective circumstances of your life. "The mind is its own place, and in itself Can make a Heaven of Hell, a Hell of Heaven", John Milton wrote in *Paradise Lost*. Philosophers, writers, and great grand-mothers of times past have long highlighted the benefits of positive thinking. While there are several ways to boost positive thinking, the expression of gratitude is an effective strategy for achieving well-being.

Gratitude is many things to many people. It is wonder; it is appreciation; it is looking at the brighter side of a setback; it is fathoming abundance; it is thanking someone in your life; it is thanking God; it is "**counting blessings**". The average person, however, probably associates gratitude with saying thank you for a gift or benefit received.

The world's most prominent researcher and writer about gratitude, Robert Emmons, defines it as "a felt sense of wonder, thankfulness, and appreciation for life". You feel grateful by noticing how fortunate your circumstances are. By definition, the practice of gratitude involves a focus on present moment, on appreciating your life as it is today and what has made it so.

Expressing gratitude is a lot more than saying thank you. Emerging research has recently shown multiple benefits. People who are consistently grateful have been found to be relatively happier, more energetic, and more hopeful. They report experiencing more frequent positive emotions. They also tend to be more helpful and empathetic, more spiritual and religious, more forgiving and less materialistic than others who are less predisposed to gratefulness. Furthermore, the more a person is inclined to gratitude, the less likely he or she is to be depressed, anxious, lonely, envious and neurotic. All these research findings are correlational; we cannot know whether being grateful causes all these good benefits or possessing good things make people grateful.

In the very first set of studies, one group of participants was asked to write down five things for which they were thankful — namely, to count their blessings — and to do so once a week for ten weeks in a row. Other groups of participants were asked to think about other five daily hassles or five major events that occurred to them. The findings were exciting. Relative to the control group, those participants counting their blessings tended to feel more optimistic and more satisfied with their lives. Even their health received a boost; they reported fewer physical symptoms.

In another study the effect of strategy of counting one's blessing was investigated. Participants were asked to keep a sort of gratitude journal – to write down and contemplate five things for which they felt grateful. The exact instructions were as follows: "There are many things in our lives, both large and small, that we might be grateful about. Think back over the events of the past week and write down on the lines below up to five things that happened for which you are grateful or thankful". Five lines followed, headed by "This week I am grateful for".

The participants were engaged in this intervention over the course of six weeks. Half of the participants were instructed to do it once a week (every Sunday night), and half to do it three times a week (every Tuesday, Thursday, and Sunday). As expected, participants involved in intervention showed greater happiness than control group participants.

There are several explanations for positive effects of counting blessings. First, grateful thinking promotes the memory and positive life experiences. By taking pleasure in some of the gifts of your life, you will be able to extract the maximum possible satisfaction and enjoyment from your current circumstances. Second, expressing gratitude bolsters self-worth and self-esteem. When you realize how much people have done for you or how much you have accomplished, you feel more confident and efficacious. Third, gratitude helps people cope with stress. Expressing gratefulness during personal adversity can help you adjust, move on and perhaps begin anew. Fourth, the expression of gratitude encourages moral behaviours. Fifth, gratitude can help build social bonds, strengthening existing relationship and nurturing new ones. Sixth, expressing gratitude tends to inhibit insidious comparisons with others. Seventh, the practice of gratitude is incompatible with negative emotions and may actually diminish or deter such feeling as anger, bitterness and greed.

Practice of Gratitude

It is advisable to practice gratitude. There are several ways. People can choose a strategy that fits with their personality and attitude.

Gratitude journal. If you enjoy writing, choose a time of day when you have several minutes to step outside your life and reflect. It may be the first thing in the morning, or during lunch, or before bedtime. Ponder the three to five things for which you are currently grateful. The events may range from the mundane (your TV set is fixed, your flowers are finally in bloom, your spouse got you a gift) to the magnificent experiences (your children received awards).

Paths to gratitude. Some of you may not enjoy writing. You may contemplate. Choose one thing each day. You may think of a particular goal and try to recollect the help and assistance you have received in the context of this goal fulfillment. This strategy would help to count your blessings in an effective manner.

Keep the strategy fresh. If you have been practicing a strategy for a long time (say, writing the events), you may become bored with the routine and may cease to extract much meaning from it. You should now change the strategy. Talk to a friend, express gratitude through art (photography, wall magazines) you may purposefully vary the mode of communicating the gratitude messages.

Direct expression. Express gratitude directly to another. The use of phones, letters, emails and face-to-face communication are recommended. Express your appreciation in concrete terms. The target persons may be your parents, favorite uncle, or old friend, old coach, teacher or supervisor. Write him or her a letter now. If possible, visit and read the letter out loud in person, on either a special day (birthday, anniversary). Describe in detail what he or she has done for you and how it has influenced your life. Some people find it uplifting to write gratitude letters to individuals whom they don't know personally.

Have you ever written letters of gratitude to your teachers / professors who have impacted your life in a significant way? Have you written letters of thankfulness to writers / poets who have made an impact on your taste and temperaments? Have you expressed gratitude to artists whose contributions you adore? *If you have not done it in the past, do it now.*

There are multiple ways to practice the strategy of gratitude, it would be wise to choose what works best for you. *Select at least one option and give it a go.* When the strategy loses its freshness or meaningfulness, don't hesitate to make a change in how, when, and how often you express yourself.

Childhood Antecedents of Self-Efficacy

Self-efficacy is a learned human pattern of thinking rather than a genetically endowed one. It begins in infancy and continues throughout the life span. Self-efficacy is based on the premise of social cognitive theory, which holds that humans actively shape their lives rather than passively reacting to environmental forces (Bandura, 1977).

The Stanford University psychologist Albert Bandura is the proponent of the construct of self-efficacy. He makes a distinction between *skill acquisition* and *skill execution*. We acquire skills through the process of going to schools/colleges, participating in the job training, and working in different sectors that offer feedback. But skill execution requires a belief system. It requires the belief that we can do the work competently (Bandura, 1977).

Bandura (1977) defines self-efficacy as the extent of belief that the person can execute a function competently. Like any other variable, it has a quantitative dimension ranging from 0 (zero) unit to 100 units. In other words, it refers to the extent of perceived capability. Drawing on Bandura's concept, a group of psychologists from Free University of Berlin have developed a psychometric measure of self-efficacy. What it measures is termed *generalized self-efficacy*.

Operationally speaking, self-efficacy may take *three* different forms: *generalized self-efficacy, domain-specific self-efficacy* and *collective self-efficacy*. The generalized self-efficacy denotes the capability belief in general. This is a trait-like concept. However, a person with a high generalized self-efficacy would not venture out to save a drowning child, since the person does not know how to swim. Obviously what is more important is the domain-specific self-efficacy. A driver should have driving efficacy and a home maker needs to have home management efficacy. This is a state-like (developable) concept. The measurement of domain-specific efficacy is very simple. An example can be offered in the extent of driving efficacy. A number of questions can be asked and the answer is possible with a reply of 'yes' or 'no'. the questions may take the following format:

"Can you drive well when the road conditions are bad? _ _ _ _ when road is very busy? _ _ _ _ when it is raining? _ _ _ _ when you are feeling feverish? _ _ _ _ when your friends are distracting you? _ _ _ _ when traffic signals are poor? _ _ _ _ when illumination level is very low? If there are fifty such questions and your 'yes' reply counts to 45, you get a score of 90 on driving efficacy. In contrast, your driving efficacy score is only 10 when you give five 'yes' answers. In this way, domain-specific efficacy scores can be determined by putting odds and asking participants to indicate the extents they can execute a function.

A number of situations require *team efficacy* or *collective efficacy*. If a new syllabus is introduced in a school, its workability and success would not depend only on the school principal or a particular teacher. It would depend collectively on the entire group of teachers. In other words, any social, cultural or organizational change is dependent on the entire school staff.

The key question in the context of self-efficacy concerns the source of self-efficacy. More specifically, the socialization parameters of self-efficacy are a critical issue. Fortunately the recent research has identified a number of childhood antecedents of self-efficacy.

Exposure to Mastery Experiences

People in general have a natural tendency to stick to their comfort zone; they seldom wish to risk their securities. So also are children. Children avoid risks. Yet an adaptive and competent mother attempts to expose her children to unusual experiences. Suppose there is a circus in the city. The mother knows that a young child would be scared of the unusual surroundings. The high voltage illumination would tire his or her senses; the high intensity drums and sound would induce fear. Despite these disturbing stimuli, an adaptive mother may say: "dear baby! Don't get scared. If you feel uncomfortable, come close to me. I would give you protection. But let us go to enjoy the circus". This is the right kind of temperament.

Parents and teachers must provide guidance. Yet children must be exposed to new experiences, new situations and unfamiliar surroundings. That's why teachers encourage students to leave the boundaries of their homes and schools to go to test their skills. They are encouraged to go elsewhere to participate in games and sports. They are advised to go to other institutions to participate in various competitions. They are inspired to accept challenges in regional and national contests. Children's tendency to expose themselves in novel situation helps them build their self-efficacy.

Guidance for Task-Selection

During the formative years of life, children and

adolescents come across a wide variety of tasks. In the beginning they do not possess adequate skills to evaluate the task difficulty. They also do not know the limits of their skills. As a result, they encounter elements of uncertainties. Sometimes they choose very easy tasks to gain cent percent success. With easy tasks, they get easy successes and become happy. But life is not a straight line. When they face slightly more difficult task and encounter failure, they become depressed.

In contrast, other category of children chooses formidable tasks in the beginning. They approach the task like gamblers. Needless to say, repeated failures induce a sense of helplessness (passivity) and hopelessness in them. They also become depressed. What is the correct approach then?

Positive psychologists suggest a balanced way of structuring the tasks. Children should start from the *tasks of moderate difficulty level*. In the beginning, attention should be focused on tasks of moderate difficulty level. Having done it successfully, children get positive feedback and their confidence is strengthened. Later they may move to perform more and more difficult work. Since children may not be having requisite skills and knowledge to assess task difficulties in all the occasions (as they do not know the limits of their skills), parents and teachers ought to provide guidance. With proper guidance, children can have right kind of *structuring of their initial tasks*. Once initial structuring is done correctly, subsequent performance is likely to be efficacious.

Role Models

Formation and change of behaviour is not limited to the provision of rewards and punishment. The observation of behaviours of others plays a very significant role in shaping human behaviours. We observe other people and get changed. We see examples and our behaviour pattern is altered. We imitate our role models and change our mindset. Role models play a very important role in building children's self-efficacy.

While *role models* are very important in shaping children's self-efficacy, a seminal point has to be delineated. Bandura (1997) has observed a subtle feature in the context of role model. The crucial question involves: Which of the role models would be imitated? A role model may be extraordinary with exceptional attributes. Yet it is found that such a role model is adored, not imitated. The reason is obvious. Although we adore the role model, we see a psychological distance. We may argue within ourselves: "This person has achieved so much in life because he comes of a noble family. Many of his friends are top-ranking individuals. He possesses a lot of wealth. But I am a struggling person. He is far away from me". This type of reasoning would create a distance between the role model and myself. Although I am inclined to honour him or her, I may not be motivated to imitate him or her. Children would also see the distance between a far-fetched role model and himself/herself.

In order to get around this problem of psychological distance, we should adopt role model from our near surroundings. For persuading children, adults (parents and teachers) must adopt children's role model from their vicinity. The case of their classmates is a good point. Parents and teachers can easily persuade a child with the example of their classmates/playmates: "If he or she done it, you can also do it. If he or she has some advantages, you have also some advantages. If you have some difficulties, he or she might be having other difficulties which you do not see". Thus, the similarity between the child and his/her role model would create a sense of similarity and the child would feel an urge to imitate. The adoption of role model from the near vicinity is a key element in the context of adult's imitation as well as child's imitation.

Once role model is identified and adopted, it would serve two essential functions. First, role model is an effective *source of information*. Observing the role model, the child can gather a lot of information. The style of conversation, the mode of doing a work, the manner of solving a problem and interactional skills can be learned through observations. Second, role model is a *source of inspiration*. Very recently a bulk of research has evidenced the motivational impact of positive emotions (Fredrickson, 2001). The psychological communion with the role model consistently inspires the child to develop and execute efficacious behaviours.

Social Persuasion

Social persuasion plays a significant role in inducing and strengthening self-efficacy. Parents and teachers need to operate at two different levels. As parents and teachers, they need to keep saying: we can do it. This kind of thinking is likely to work at a neurological level to cement self-confidence of parents and teachers.

Parents and teachers also need to keep saying to children: "you can do it". The constant repetition of this mantra "you can do it" would be immensely helpful for children. The exposure of children to such social persuasion would trigger self-thinking in the positive direction.

Positive Interpretation of Arousal

It is a natural phenomenon that prolonged intensive

activity generates negative physiological signals. We get fatigued when we work for a long period. The fatigue, tiredness and monotony are all outcomes of prolonged physical activities. Yet, how we interpret these negative signals makes a difference. If we interpret it in a negative way, we stop working and give up efforts. But our positive interpretation of these negative signals keeps us going.

Parents and teachers need to train children to use positive interpretation of physiological arousal. If they learn to attach meaning to arousal indicators, their motivation level would not decline, rather they would stay invigorated.

In sum, self-efficacy is a very dynamic process to activate cognitive, affective and motivational resources in children. The sources of childhood antecedents of self-efficacy can be tapped by exposing children to mastery experiences, helping children to start working from tasks of moderately difficult level, providing right kind of role models from the vicinity, by using social persuasion, and guiding children to interpret physiological arousal in a meaningful way (Sahoo, 2015).

■

References

Bandura, A. (1977). Self-efficacy: Toward a unifying theory of behavioral change. *Psychological Review*, 84, 191-215.

Bandura, A. (1997). *Self-efficacy: The exercise of control*. New York: W.H. Freeman.

Fredrickson, B.L. (2001). The broaden-and-build theory of positive emotions. *American Psychologist*, 56, 218-226.

Sahoo, F.M. (2015). *Mind management*. Bhubaneswar ASHRA Publication.

Flow: Mechanism of Living in the Present

The present moment is all we are really guaranteed. Enjoying this present moment is a surer way of attaining peace and happiness. Flow is a state of intense absorption and involvement with the present moment. Have you ever been absorbed in what you were doing – painting, writing, conversing, fishing, playing chess, praying, web-surfing – that you completely lost track of time? Perhaps you failed to notice that you were very hungry or your back ached from sitting for so long? Did nothing else seem to matter? If the answer is yes, then you have experienced a state called flow.

Coined by a psychologist, Mihaly Csikeszentmihalyi, flow denotes a state of complete absorption in what one is doing. You are totally immersed in what you are doing, fully concentrating, and unaware of yourself. The activity you are performing is challenging and engrossing stretching your skills and experience. When in flow, people report feeling strong and efficacious, at the peak of their abilities, alert, in control, and completely unselfconscious. They do the activity for the sheer sake of doing it.

Csikszentmihalyi argued that the good life, a happy life is characterized by flow, by "complete absorption in what one does". The key to creating flow is to establish a balance between skills and challenge. Whether you are rockclimbing, performing surgery, writing a story or driving on the highway, if the challenges of the situation overwhelm your level of skill or expertise, you will feel anxious or frustrated. On the other hand, if the activity is not challenging enough, you will become bored. Flow is a way of describing your experience that falls in just the right space between boredom and anxiety. Your happiness depends on your ability to find the perfect space, to extract flow from what you are doing. The situation can be depicted schematically.

		Perceived Ability	
		Low	High
Level of challenge in task	High	Anxiety	Flow
	Low	Apathy	Boredom

Benefits of Flow

Flow is inherently pleasurable and fulfilling. The enjoyment one obtains is generally lasting and reinforcing. Flow provides a natural high that, unlike artificial highs or hedonic pleasures, is a positive, productive and controllable experience that does not cause guilt or shame.

Second, because flow states are intrinsically rewarding, we naturally want to repeat them. However, there lies a seeming paradox. As we master new skills, our experience of flow diminish because the task at hand is no longer as stimulating. Thus, to maintain flow, we continually have to test ourselves in ever more challenging activities. We have to apply focused mental discipline in ever more challenging activities. We have to stretch our skill or find novel opportunities to use them. This is wonderful, because we are constantly striving, growing, learning and becoming more competent, expert, and complex.

One of the core ideas connected with flow experience is that we cannot allow our happiness to depend on our external circumstances, for every positive event and accomplishment we experience are accompanied by rapid adaptation and escalating expectations. Even as we attain great heights, we begin to want even more. There is no inherent problem in our desire to escalate our goals, as long as we enjoy the struggle along the way.

The experience of flow leads us to be involved in life (rather than be alienated from it), to enjoy activities (rather than to find them dreary), to have a sense of control (rather than helplessness), and to feel a strong sense of self (rather than unworthiness). All these factors imbue life with meaning and lend it a richness and intensity.

Increasing Flow Experience

Flow opens up to a world of a very different kind, a world of thousand possibilities and opportunities. Finding flow involves the ability to expand your mind and body to its limits, to strive to accomplish something difficult, novel, or worthwhile, and to discover rewards in the process of each moment, indeed in life itself.

Control attention. To increase the frequency and length of flow experience in your daily life, you need to become fully involved and engaged. Whether it is writing a letter, doing a job-related task, or undertaking leisure activities that engage your skills and expertise. How exactly do you accomplish that? The secret is **attention**. William James, the 'father' of psychology once wrote: "*My experience is what I agree to attend to*". This is a revolutionary thought.

What you notice and what you pay attention to is your experience; it is your life. There is only so much attention that you have go around, so how and where you choose to invest it is critical. To enter the state of flow, attention needs to be directed fully to the task at hand. When you're intensely concentrating on doing something, you're essentially directing your attention to the task (e.g., writing poems as opposed to other activities like deciding about breakfast and inquiry about time).

Maintaining the state of flow also involves the control of your attention. If the challenge is too low you become bored; your attention drifts to some other thing. If the challenge is too high, you become self-conscious. Your aim is to gain control over what you pay attention to. Hence choose contents of your task wisely.

Adopt new values. Happy people have the capacity to enjoy their lives even when their material conditions are lacking and even when many of their goals have not been reached. How do they do it? They follow certain paths. They are open to new and different values (cooking, playing, etc). Thy learn until the day they die. The state of flow comes naturally to the child, but we may have to work at it.

Learn what flows. Many people believe that the conditions of work and task always generate stress while no-work condition affords pleasure. This is a wrong idea. There are many studies to show that people have negative thoughts when they are not doing anything. Hence it would be proper to select and choose activity that suits you and affords flow. With an open mind, search the task that has potential for flow experience.

Transform routine tasks. Even seemingly boring and tedious activities – waiting for the train, listening to a dull presentation – can be transformed into something more meaningful and stimulating – what you need to do is to create microflow activities with specific goals. For example, you could solve problems in your head, tap melodies to favourite songs. So, when you sit in a doctor's waiting room, your goal might be to draw a project design.

Flow in conversation. Depending on your job and lifestyle, a significant percentage of your days may be spent in conversation with others. Do you usually experience flow when you are talking with another person? Focus your attention as intensely as possible on what the other person is saying and your reaction to his words. Do not be too quick to respond, rather, give him the space to expand on his thoughts. You may prompt him with brief follow-up questions (And then what happened? And Why did you think so?)

Smart work. One fascinating study of work found that people tend to use their work as one of three ways: as a job, as a career, or as a calling. Those who place their work in the job category essentially perceive it as a necessary evil, a means to an end – the job is needed to support them. People who report having career may see their work as means for promoting their status. Those who see their work as calling report enjoy work and find it to be fulfilling and socially useful. It is important to recognize that people regarding their work as a calling are likely to experience flow during their work process.

While discussing different possibilities of flow experience, a caveat needs to be identified. In the process of experiencing flow, some individuals can become addict; they may ignore their primary responsibility. However, with the use of human intelligence and discrimination, people can guard against this addictive practice. Once this caveat is recognized, seeking flow experience is likely to be a source of good life, happy life. ■

Savouring: An Alternative for Living in the Present

The ability to savour the positive experiences in your life is one of the most important ingredients of happiness. Most people truly understand what it means to savour after overcoming uncomfortable or painful symptoms. When you have a toothache and it's gone, you suddenly delight in its absence. When you are overwhelmed by terrible allergies that abruptly dissipate, you truly relish breathing freely.

You can think of savouring as having a past, present, and future component. You savour the past by remembering about the good old days – your wedding, your appointment letter, and your pleasant vacation. You savour the present by wholly living in, being mindful of and relishing the present moment, whether it's having lunch with a friend, immersed yourself in a book, song, or project at work. This type of savouring overlaps a great deal with flow. Finally you savour the future by anticipating and fantasizing about upcoming positive events. This is an element of optimistic thinking. Although it may appear that the past and future components of savouring are not included in the process of "living in the present", both involve ways of bringing and preserving pleasure of the past and future into the present moment.

Researchers define savouring as the thoughts or behaviors capable of "generating, intensifying, and prolonging enjoyment". When you stop and smell the roses instead of walking by, you are savouring. When you bask and take pride in your own or friend's accomplishment, you are savouring. There is slight difference between flow and savouring. Savouring requires a stepping outside of experience and reviewing it (e.g., how beautiful is the rose), whereas flow involves a complete immersion in experience.

Strategies to Foster Savouring

If savouring life's joy is one powerful activity for sustainable happiness, people need to use available options to trigger savouring. Anyone can select an option and get started right now.

Relish ordinary experiences. The first challenge in using the strategy of savouring is to learn how to appreciate and take pleasure in mundane everyday experiences. Consider as a model what participants were asked to do in recent research aimed at exploring the extent to which making savouring a habit can produce tangible benefits. In one set of studies, depressed participants were invited to take a few minutes once a day to relish something that they usually hurry through (e.g., eating a meal, taking a shower). When it was over they were instructed to write down in what ways they had experienced the event differently as well as how that felt compared with the times when they rushed through it.

Starting tomorrow, consider your daily routine activity and ritual. Do you notice and savour the pleasure of the day, or do you dash through them? If the latter, then resolve to seize the pleasures when they happen and take full advantage of them. Linger over your morning breakfast or afternoon snack, absorbing the aroma, the sweetness (rather than mindlessly consuming). Strive to bask in the feeling of accomplishment when you have finished a task at home or work, rather than distractedly moving on to the next item on your to-do list. Enjoy the little thing, for one day you may look back and realize they were the big things.

Savour and reminisce with family and friends. Often it is easier to savour when you share a positive experience with another. Whether you have visited an interesting place or listening to an inspiring speech, the pleasure of the moment can be heightened to the company of others who similarly value the experience. You might reminisce together about a party you both attended or a vacation you shared. The advantage of savouring and reminiscing with friends and family members bring abundant positive emotions.

Transport yourself. The ability to engage in positive reminiscence – to transport yourself at will to a different place and time – can provide both pleasure and solace when you need it most. People can travel to mental destinations through recall of positive images and memories. People make lists of happy memories and personal memories (such as photographs, gifts and souvenirs) and then engage in positive memories.

Replay happy days. The practice of repetitively replaying your happy life events serves to prolong and reinforce positive emotions. So think about one of your happiest days – the first day of your school, the first day your child called you papa / mama. Replay it in your mind as though you were rewinding a videotape and playing it back. Think about the events of the day, and remember what happened in as much detail as you can.

Celebrate good news. Sharing successes and accomplishments with others has been shown to be associated with elevated pleasant emotions and well-being. So, when you or your spouse or cousin or friend wins an honour, congratulate him or her (and yourself), and celebrate. Try to enjoy the occasion to the fullest. Passing on and rejoicing in good news lead you to relish and soak up the present moment, as well as to foster connections with others.

Be open to beauty and excellence. The strategy involves allowing yourself to truly admire an object of beauty or display talent, genius, or virtue. Strive even to feel reverence and awe. Positive psychologists suggest that people who open themselves to the beauty and excellence around them are more likely to find joy, meaning, and profound connections in their lives.

Be mindful. Many philosophical and spiritual traditions stress the cultivation of mindfulness as a critical ingredient of well-being. The practice of Zen Buddhism, for example, emphasizes clearing one's mind and grounding oneself in the present moment. A series of studies conducted at the University of Rochester focused on people high in mindfulness – that is, those who are prone to be mindfully attentive to the *here and now and keenly aware of their surroundings*. These people with practice of mindfulness exhibit greater well-being.

Take pleasure in the senses. Pay close attention to and take delight in momentary pleasures, wonders, and magical moments. Focus on the sweetness of a ripe mango, the aroma of a bakery, or the warmth of the sun when you step out from the shade. Take in the cool fresh air after a storm, the brushstrokes of a painting.

Create a savouring album. You may take snaps when

you travel. Collect pictures that are likely to give you happiness. Preserve the savouring album and see through the pictures whenever you feel like savouring.

A note about writing. Some psychologists advise savouring through writing, perhaps by keeping a journal in which you describe a memorable past experience or an exciting time in the present. Since writing is a structured activity, some people may not find it very pleasant. Yet, some people may find it to be useful.

Thinking of good times from the past makes you feel better about the present. It helps you appreciate things more. It gives you an idea of where I was then, where I am now and where I ultimately want to be. These memories also give you confidence: "I did it before, I can do it again".

Preventing Negative Changes Related to Aging

Throughout the world, better health procedures have led to an increasing life expectancy. With individuals living longer, there is also a greater choice of developing neurocognitive disorder such as Alzheimer and Parkinson's. Within the same age-group mortality is higher for people with neurocognitive disorders than for those without.

Two consistent findings are that older adults show changes in brain structure and that they use their brains in different ways from younger adults. In terms of brain volume, volume reduction is seen on the *hippocampus, cerebellum, prefrontal cortex (PFC),* and *caudate nucleus,* which are areas related to executive functions and memory. The visual cortex and the entorhinal cortex show little reduction in volume with age. The entorhinal cortex is located in the temporal lobe and serves as a hub that connects the hippocampus and the neocortex. It is involved in memory and spatial navigation. It is one of the first areas affected in Alzheimer's disorder.

In order to solve problems, older individuals use their brains differently. Even when younger and older adults both perform a memory task successfully, the older adults recruit more brain regions than do younger adults.

As you are sitting and doing nothing, the **default network** in your brain turns on. When you start performing a task, more task-related networks are activated and the default network is inhibited. In younger individuals the same pattern of activity in the frontal lobes, the parietal lobes, the temporal lobes and the cingulated is seen across a variety of tasks. In older individuals, the number of brain areas involved in the default network is larger, especially in the frontal lobes. Older adults also have a more difficult time turning off the default network. It is assumed that this is related to the problems some older adults have in shifting cortical resources to new tasks.

Can an individual's activities be protective in brain changes? The answer to this question is **yes**. It was first noticed that not all individuals show the same changes to similar neurocognitive disorders or brain injury. From this observation, the concept of **reserve** was developed. That is, high functioning individuals tend to show less loss of cognitive abilities in relation to neurocognitive disorders. The concept of reserve suggests that the brain can compensate for problems in neural functioning. In high functioning individuals, brains of older individuals expand their networks to solve problems. High functioning or intelligence is often associated with greater reserve.

Additional research has shown a role for exercise and social support. Exercise is thought to play an important role in aging by promoting healthy cardiovascular function. That is, exercise increases blood flow to the entire brain. Exercise has also been shown to slow its expression of Alzheimer disorder. Exercise provides multiple routes in enhancing cognitive vitality across the life span. Those include the reduction of disease risk as well as improvement in molecular and cellular structures of the brain. This, in turn, increases brain function. Further, it is suggested that aerobic exercise affects executive functions more than other cognitive processes.

Social support has also been associated with a reduced risk for neurocognitive disorders. Two of these factors are the size of one's network of friends and whether one is married or not. As suggested in studies of the social brain, understanding and maintaining network of friends require a variety of cognitive resources which in turn offer a reserve for dealing with brain pathologies. One study followed 16,638 individuals over the age of 50 for 6 years. Those individuals who were more socially integrated and active showed less memory loss during the 6-year period.

Social Brain

Our present-day emotionality has largely evolved within a social context. In terms of brain structure, many of the structures involved in the processing of emotion are important. Brain structure involved in social interactions can be recognized in terms of three processes.

The first process involves higher-level neurocortical regions in the processing of sensory information. This is how we know who we experience through vision, hearing, touch and other sensory processes. Research suggests when looking at a face, we process broad categorization related to gender and to the emotion expressed before we complete the detailed construction of the entire face and determine who we are seeing.

Second, our affect system will help us predict what people will do socially. As we see a social interaction, what happens on the level of the brain? What happens first involves the amygdale striatum and orthofrontal cortex. The amygdale is involved in processing the emotional significance of the event. This includes positive emotions such as a person you care about smiling at you as well as negative emotions such as seeing someone angry or fearful. Activation also takes place if a person looks untrustworthy. This determination occurs independent of gender, race, eye gaze, or emotionality expressed. Through its connection with other areas, the amygdale also can influence memory, attention, and decision making. Overall, these areas help us know the emotional context of our perception and what we need to do about them.

The third process involves the higher cortical regions of the neocortex. These regions are involved in cognitive understanding and regulation. These are the areas that let us construct an inner model of our social world. Included in this model would be some social understanding of others, their relationship with us are the meaning of our action for them. It is these areas that are most likely associated with theory of mind, our ability to attribute mental states to other people. Indeed, damage to the orthofrontal cortex does reduce our ability to detect a faux pas in a given situation.

The prefrontal cortex has also been shown to be activated during humour, social – norm transgressions resulting in embarrassment, and moral emotions. With damage to this area, individuals have difficulty knowing that another person is being deceptive. We have not only evolved systems for determining basic emotions such as fear, joy or anger, but also for the most socially related ones, such as guilt, embarrassment, jealousy, and pride.

The prefrontal cortex appears to be involved in various aspects of social relationships, social cooperation, moral behavior, and social aggression. Overall, sensory information is processed by sensory cortex, its emotional value is determined by structures such as the amygdale, and the social implications determined by the prefrontal cortex.

Using fMRI research, brain processes involved in the variety of tasks required for social interactions have been identified. The social brain can be seen as composed of areas involved in the detection of social processes including face recognition (the fusiform face area, FFA), emotional recognition (the amygdale, insula, anterior cingulated cortex, ACC), and regulating cognitive processes involving the frontal areas of the brain.

Preference for human faces begins shortly after birth in humans. As the child matures, cortical areas such as the FFS in the temporal lobe show greater differentiation. Through its connection comes the ability to recognize and remember faces, which continues into adulthood. Individuals with autism spectrum disorder do not focus on the faces – especially the eyes – of others. Increased differentiation of emotional facial expressions involves the amygdale. Interestingly enough, adolescents show greater reactivity of emotional faces than adults.

Storytelling: The Style that Works in Leadership Talks

Leadership communication, in order to be effective, needs to build a relationship between people. A trusted leader who communicates with integrity can develop relationship of trust with people all over the organization, even with those whom she has never met. It has been recently found that the art of storytelling is a powerful glue that binds the leader to people.

Good stories are influential. Great ones inspire cultures and beliefs. Inspirational leaders are often called great storytellers. Stories are easily memorable, as they follow the pattern used by the brain to lay down episodic memories, with a timeline – beginning, middle and end. If a story is consistent with what our brain expects, coherent and plausible, it can be more persuasive than the truth. Our brains are consistently using past patterns to predict the future. When the future doesn't fit with what we expect we experience dissonance or discomfort. A story that fits with the expected patterns keeps us in the comfort zone. Equally, our brains are always searching for meaning, for a cause to an observed effect, for a purpose for an action. A story that gives plausible reasons and causes tends to be believed.

A story is a whole, and one part might trigger others, thus making it more memorable and easily re-tellable. Some call the capacity to be easily retold part of "conversational capital". Some stories appear to be fundamental or archetypical, like myths, and in the telling and multiple retelling help shape the values and culture of the community or organization. For example, the great start-up story where the founders of the organization were young, experienced great hardship and were misunderstood but worked all hours were creative geniuses, stayed true to themselves, and the great benefits their product – simpler, better designed, more usable – brought to the world, and made the company into a globe success.

There is evidence that in reading or listening to stories, our brains mirror some of the activities of the agents in the story, for example smell words cause our olfactory system to fire, actions our mirror neurons, emotions our emotional networks.

A story that makes sense of a chaotic, complex environment enables staff to perform better because it lessens the brain's fear of uncertainty and the discomfort caused by ambiguity. It creates a good feeling, due to the ease with which the brain accepts what the story is telling.

There is some evidence that reading a lot of factors improves our ability to empathize with others, and improves our social awareness, implying that the mirroring leads to empathizing with the actors in stories, as we do with the real people in our lives. If a leader tells a great, plausible story about themselves, with emotions, which reveals values that are common to a majority of listeners, they can resonate with the "hero" and it creates a kind of relationship.

■

What's Ahead

Our orientation to time affects positive and negative outcomes alike. Although we may have a rough idea about how much time we spend thinking about the future, it is useful to reflect to produce an estimate of the time spent "in the past", "in the present", and "in the future".

We can mark a piece of lined paper with columns and rows (see below). From the top down in each column, we may write the hours of our day (7 am, 8 am, 9 am …..) and across the top in a row write the words *Past*, *Present*, and *Future*. Now we have a chart on which we can write how many *minutes* in each hour were spent to thoughts of the past, present or future.

Time	Past	Present	Future
7 am			
8 am			
9 am			
10 am			
11 am			
-			
-			
-			
-			
10 pm			
Totals			

It helps us to draw some inferences about our time orientation. It is possible to estimate the number of minutes one spends in each of the columns.

It is important to note that there is no right or wrong ways to spend our time. Instead, the purpose is to sensitize us to the temporal loci of our thinking. Ofcourse, the results of this exercise may depend on the day of the week, our health, our age, whether we are on vacation, the time of the year, where we live, our job, and so on.

There are advantages and disadvantages to each of the three temporal orientations – the past, the present, the future. Let us begin with the past orientation. It is mostly characterized by an emphasis on pleasurable views of previous interpersonal relationships with friends and family. This sentimental perspective focuses on the happiness to be derived in warm personal interactions. However, there is no guarantee that the view of the past is positive; those who hold negative views about their past are filled with ruminations, anxieties, and depressive thoughts and feelings. Assessment of use of this orientation, must be viewed from within a cultural lens, however for example, from a Western perspective, the past orientation can produce a very conservative, overly cautious approach to one's life, along with a desire to preserve the status quo that makes the person unwilling to experience new things. From an Eastern perspective, however, paying attention to the past might ensure safe passage of tradition and ritual from generation to generation.

Now, let us explore the person who lives in the here and now. The person who lives for the present can be described in hedonistic terms that have both good and bad consequences. Living in the moment, this individual derives great pleasure in highly intensive activities, relishes the thrills and excitement found in the here and now, and remains open to the ongoing adventures of the moment. The person focused on the present also may place a premium on excitement.

One aspect of enjoying the ongoing experience can be savouring (recollection of sweet memories). Although savouring can be applied to the past or the future, one of the most robust types of savouring pertains to the enjoyment of the moment, perhaps even acting to stretch out an ongoing positive event.

When considered from a Western perspective, the concerns that arise from the present orientation all reflect the fact that such a person may not think ahead about the potential liabilities of such excitement seeking. When adults are solely committed to this present orientation, some may suffer the negative consequences of hedonistic adventures. For example, addiction, injuries from accident and various temptations can destroy the career aspirations. Much of the negative consequences of the present orientation have distinctively Western flavour. An Eastern perspective would include a meditative appreciation of the calmness that flows from a here-and-now orientation. If one considers a more Eastern perspective, many of these negative consequences are less likely to appear (if they appear at all).

Finally, there is the future temporal perspective. The person with a future orientation thinks ahead to the possible consequences of his or her actions. Such persons have clear goals and conjure the requisite paths to reach these goals. They are likely to engage in preventive behavior to lessen the likelihood of bad things happening in future. Furthermore, these individuals develop self-confidence (self-efficacy), optimism and hope that lead them to success in various domains of life (academics, sports, jobs, health and social activities).

In reading about the past, the present, and the future, one may be intrigued about which orientation should characterize our lives. The key to having a balance in these three temporal perspectives is our ability to operate in the temporal orientation that best fits the situation in which we find ourselves. This balance entails, "Working hard when it's time to work. Playing intensively when it's time to play. Enjoying listening to grandma's old stories while she is still alive. **Being flexible and capable of switching to an appropriate time orientation yields the most productive approach to how we spend our time**. Although Western culture typically emphasizes future orientation, an intelligent transition from one mode to the other appears to be the wisest choice.

Gratitude

The term *gratitude* is derived from the Latin concept gratia, which entails some variant of grace, gratefulness, and graciousness. The ideas flowing from the Latin root pertain to kindness, generousness, gifts, the beauty of giving and receiving. In the words of noted University of California researcher Robert Emmons (2005), gratitude emerges upon recognizing that one has obtained a positive outcome from another individual who behaved in a way that was 1) costly to him or her, 2) valuable to the recipient, and 3) intentionally rendered. As such, gratitude taps into the propensity to appreciate and savour everyday events and experience.

In Emmon's definition, the positive outcome appears to have come from another person; however, the benefit may be derived from a nonhuman's action or event. For example, the individual who has undergone a traumatic natural event such a family member's survival of a cyclone feels a profound sense of gratitude. In a related vein, it has been suggested that events of larger magnitude also should produce higher levels of gratitude. Researchers have reasoned that gratitude should be greater when the giving person's actions are judged praiseworthy and when they deviate positively from that which was expected.

Gratitude is viewed as a prized human propensity in

all religions. Not only is gratitude seen as beneficial to the individual, but it also serves as a motivational force for human altruism.

Cultivating Gratitude

Charles Dickens writes: "Reflect on your present blessings, of which every man has many, not on your past misfortunes of which all men have some". There are various ways to enhance the sense of gratitude. Gratitude journal is an effective method. People can keep weekly gratitude journal to record events for which people were grateful. Those who keep gratitude journals report greater enthusiasm, alertness, and determination. They are significantly more likely to make progress towards important goals pertaining to their health, interpersonal relationship, and academic performances. Indeed, those who are in the "**count your blessings**" diary condition also are more likely to have helped another person. Furthermore, people in gratitude condition (*maintaining a diary that records help given to other people and help received from other people on daily basis*) are more optimistic, more energetic, more connected to other people, and more likely to have restful sleep.

Other researchers have shown that positive traits have been associated with self-reported gratitude. Adolescents who count their blessings have more optimism and life satisfaction and have lower experience of negative affect. In addition, feeling grateful is strongly associated with positive feelings about school experiences.

A Japanese form of meditation known as Naikan enhances a person's sense of gratitude. Using Naikan, one learns to meditate daily on three gratitude related questions: First, what did I receive? Second, what did I give? And third, what troubles and difficulties did I cause to others? Gratitude meditation helps to bring this awareness.

The effectiveness of gratitude interventions may be moderated by the level of positive affect in our lives. Some researchers asked a sample of children and adolescents to write a letter of thanks to someone for whom they were grateful and then deliver that letter in person. They then compared youth in their study who were high in positive affect with those that were low in positive affect in terms of the effectiveness of the gratitude exercise. Results showed that those youth who were low in positive affect were able to make greater increases in their levels of gratefulness and had higher positive affect post intervention. Thus, gratitude may be even more important to cultivate in individuals who are lower in regular positive emotional experience.

Measuring Gratitude
Several researches have been taken to measure gratitude. One tactic is to ask people to list things about which they feel grateful (*Gallup Poll*). This simple method allows to find those events that produce gratefulness. Another strategy is to take the stories people write about their lives and code these vignetts for gratefulness themes.

Some attempts have been made to measure gratitude behaviourally. For example, the frequency of saying "thank you" may be taken as a measure of gratitude.

Working in the context of an an overall index called the Multidimensional Prayer Inventory, researchers have developed a 3-item Thanksgiving self-report scale on which people respond along a 7-point response set (1= never to 7= All of the time) to each of them. The three Thanksgiving items are "I offered thanks for specific things", "I expressed my appreciation for my circumstances", and "I thanked

God for things occurring in my life". This scale is worded in terms of religious prayer, and higher scores have been correlated with stronger religious practices such as prayer.

The trait self-report index that appears to be most promising is the Gratitude Questionnaire (GQ) developed by Emmons and his associates. The GQ is a 6-item questionnaire (see Appendix) on which respondents endorse each item on a 7-point Likert scale (1= strongly disagree to 7= strongly agree). Scores on the GQ relate in predictable ways to other positive psychological constructs (positive emotions, vitality, optimism, hope, satisfaction with life). Moreover, it is positively associated with empathy, sharing, forgiving, and giving one's time for the benefit of others. Furthermore, those who score higher on gratitude are less concerned with material goods, and they are more likely to engage in prayer and spiritual matters.

Gratitude Questionnaire

Instruction: Using the scale below write a number beside each statement to indicate how much you agree with it.

1	2	3	4	5	6	7
Strongly Disagree	Disagree	Slightly Disagree	Neutral	Slightly Agree	Agree	Strongly Agree

1. I have so much in life to be thankful for.
2. If I had so list everything that I felt grateful for, it would be a long list.
3. When I look at the world, I don't see much to be grateful for.
4. I am grateful to a wide variety of people.
5. As I get older, I find myself more able to appreciate the people, events and situations

that have been part of my life history.

6. Long amount of time can go by before I feel grateful to something/someone.

Interpretation: Items 3 and 6 are reverse scored. (Assign score '7' for your rating of '1'; score 6
for your rating of '2' and so on)

    Add your ratings across 6 items
    Below 10: Low   20 to 30: High
    11 to 20: moderate   Above 30: very high

Expanding the Contours of Pleasure

The potency and potentialities of **positive emotions** is an important mechanism of leveraging human happiness. Cornell University psychologist Alice Isen is a pioneer in the examination of positive emotions. Isen found that, when experiencing mild positive emotions, we are more likely (1) to help other people, (2) to be flexible in our thinking, and (3) to come up with solution to our problems.

Isen contrived situations where people would successfully get changed coins by operating a machine or they would lose their inserted coin. Thus, one group of people would experience pleasure and the other group would feel sad because of the lost coin. Then the researcher measured helping behavior of people. The researcher measured whether or not people are picking up the dropped letters (with address indicated on the envelope) and post them altruistically. Results indicated that people experiencing positive emotions are doing it more often.

In another intervention, Isen examined whether or not feeling positive emotions is helping to see problem solving options for good decision making. The researcher randomly assigned physicians to an experimental condition in which the doctor either was or was not given a small bag that contained sweets (the doctors were not allowed to eat sweets during the experiment). Those physicians who had, rather than had not, been given the gift of sweets displayed superior reasoning and decision making relative to the physicians who did not receive the gift. The vignettes of the doctors' decision making process were given to independent raters to judge the efficacy of decision.

Building on Isen's work Fredrickson (2000) has developed an interesting framework, the **broaden-and-build model** that may provide some explanations for the robust social and cognitive effects of positive emotional experiences.

In testing her model, Fredrickson (2000) demonstrated that the experience of joy expands the realm of individual's ongoing activity. She involved five equitable groups of participants and used five 30-minute film clips for those five groups to induce five emotions (joy, contentment, anger, fear, or a neutral condition). Following equitable exposures, all participants were brought back to the original venue and they were offered a plain sheet of paper. The researcher promised that they would be given the opportunity of fulfilling their wishes. They were asked to write on a sheet of paper the specific things they would like to do. It was shown that participants experiencing negative emotions (anger & fear) indicated a few things whereas participants experiencing positive emotions (joy, contentment) gave a long list. Those participants who experienced joy or contentment listed significantly more desired possibilities than did the people in the neutral or negative conditions. In turn, those expanded possibilities for future activities should lead the joyful individuals to initiate subsequent activities. Those who expressed more negative emotions, on the other hand tended to shut down their thinking about subsequent possibilities. Joy appears to open us up to many new thoughts and behaviours.

Joy also increases our likelihood by behaving positively towards other people, developing more positive relationships. Furthermore, joy induces playfulness, which is quite important because such behaviours are evolutionarily adaptive in acquisition of necessary resources. Play builds (1) enduring social and intellectual resource by encouraging attachment (2) higher levels of creativity, and (3) brain development.

It appears that positive emotions build resources. Fredrickson found that people's positive emotions were instrumental in broad-minded coping (solving problems with creative means) on two occasions 5 weeks apart. The researcher found that initial levels of positive emotions predicted overall increases in creative problem solving. In sum, positive emotions such as joy may help greater resources, maintain a sense of vital energy (more positive energy), and create even more resources. Fredrickson refers to this positive sequence as the **upward spiral of** positive emotions.

Extending her model of positive emotions, Fredrickson examines the **undoing potential of positive emotions**. She suggested the ratio of positive to negative emotional experiences is associated with human flourishing. It is suggested that, given the broadening and building effects of positive emotions, joy and contentment might function as antidotes to negative emotions. To test this, the researcher exposed all participants to a situation that aroused negative emotion and immediately randomly assigned people to emotion conditions (sparked by evocative video clips) ranging from mild joy to sadness, cardiovascular recovery represented the undoing process and was operationalized as the time that elapsed from the start of the randomly assigned video until the physiological reactions induced by the initial negative emotion returned to baseline. The undoing prediction was supported, as the participants in the joy and contentment conditions were able to undo the effects of the negative emotions more quickly than the people in the other conditions.

Given that positive emotions help people build enduring resources and recover from negative resources, Fredrickson and Losada (2005) hypothesized that positive emotions might be associated with optimal mental health or flourishing. Researchers find that a mean ratio of 2:9 positive to negative emotions predict human flourishing.

Positive emotions have other benefits as well. Sonja Lyubomirsky (2006) found that success and other beneficial outcomes are caused by the presence of happiness in a person's life.

Living a Pleasurable Life

Buddha left home in search of a more meaningful existence and ultimately found enlightenment, a sense of peace and happiness. Aristotle believed that *eudaimonia* (human flourishing associated with living a life of virtue), or happiness based on a lifelong pursuit of meaningful, developmental goals (doing what is what is worth doing), was the key to the good life. These age-old definitions of happiness, along with many other conceptualizations of emotional well-being, have had clear influences on the views of the 20th and 21st century scholars, but move recent psychological theory and genetic research has helped us to clarify happiness and its correlates.

Theories of happiness have been divided into three types: (1) need / goal satisfaction theories, (2) process / activity theories, and (3) genetic / personality disposition.

In regard to need/goal satisfaction theories, the leaders of particular schools of psychotherapy posited these ideas about happiness. For example, psychoanalytic and humanistic theorists (Sigmund Freud and Abraham Maslow, respectively) suggested that the reduction of tension or satisfaction of needs lead to happiness. In short, it was believed that we are happy because we have reached our goals. Such "happiness as satisfaction" makes happiness a target of our psychological pursuits.

In the process/activity camps, theorists posit that engaging in particular life activities generates happiness. For example, Mike Csikszeritmihalyi (pronounced CHEEK-SENT-ME-HIGH), who was one of the first 20th-century scientists to examine process/activity conceptualization of happiness, proposed that people who experience flow (engagement in interesting activities that match or challenge task-related skills) in daily life tend to be very happy. Indeed, his research suggests that engagement in activity *produces* happiness. Other process/activity theorists (Emmons, Snyder) have emphasized how the *process* of pursuing goals generate energy and happiness.

Those who emphasize the genetic and personality predisposition theories of happiness (Diener) tend to see happiness as stable, whereas process/activity theorists view happiness as changing with life conditions. On this point, Costa and McCrae found that happiness changed little over a 6-year period, thereby lending credence to theories of personality-based as biologically determined happiness. More recent research, however, found evidence that the links between personality and happiness may be more idiographic than previously thought. Individuals may vary to the type of adaptation to positive or negative external experiences (Diener). In addition, these researches believe that multiple set points for positive emotion may exist for any one individual, and these set points may be able to be changed under some conditions.

Further elucidating the link between happiness and personality, researchers have showed that extroversion and neuroticism, two of the Big Five Factors of personality (openness, conscientiousness, extroversion, agreeableness, neuroticism), are closely related to the characteristics of happiness.

Studies of biological or genetic determination of happiness have found that up to 40% of positive emotionality and 55% of negative emotionality are genetically based (Tellegen). Obviously this leaves about 50% of the variance in happiness that is not explained by biological components.

Building on a utilitarian tradition and the tenets of hedonic psychology (which emphasizes the study of pleasure and life satisfaction), Diener considers well-being to be the subjective evaluation of one's current status in the world. More specifically, well-being involves our experience of pleasure and our appreciation of life's rewards. Given this view, Diener defines subjective well-being (SWB) as a combination of positive affect (in the absence of negative affect) and general life satisfaction. Furthermore, he *uses the term subjective well-being as a synonym for happiness*. (The satisfaction component is measured with *Diener's Satisfaction With Life Scale*.)

Psychologists who support the hedonistic perspective view psychological well-being and happiness as synonymous. Alternatively, scholars whose ideas about well-being are more consistent with Aristotle's views on *eudaimonia* believe that happiness and well-being are not synonymous. In this latter perspective, *eudaimonia* is composed of happiness and meaning. Stated in a simple formula,

Well-being = Meaning + Happiness

In order to subscribe to this latter view, one must understand virtue and the social implications of daily behaviour. Furthermore, this view implies that those who seek well-being be authentic and live according to their real needs and desired goals. Thus, living a eudaimonic life goes beyond experiencing "things pleasurable", and it embraces flourishing as the goal in all our actions. Both hedonistic and eudaimonic versions of happiness have influenced the 21st –century definition.

21st Century Definition

The evolved definition of happiness emphasizes pleasure, satisfaction and life meaning. Indeed, the type of happiness addressed in much of today's lives emphasizes hedonics, meaning and authenticity. For example, Seligman (2002) suggests that a pleasant and meaningful life can be built on the happiness that results from using our psychological strengths.

Describing this new model of happiness, Lyubomirsky proposes that a person's chronic happiness level is governed by three major factors: a genetically determined set point for happiness, happiness-relevant circumstantial factors and happiness-relevant activities and practices. She further states that genetics account for 50% of variance for happiness, whereas the circumstances (both good and bad) accounts for 10% of the happiness. This model leaves room for volition and self-generated goals to the tune of 40% for the attainment of pleasure, meaning and good health. Lyubomirsky stresses **intentional activities** for attainment of well-being.

Increasing Happiness in Our Life

- Realize that enduring happiness doesn't come from success. People adapt to changing circumstances.
- Take control of your time. Happy people feel control of their lives. Master the use of time. It helps to set goals and break them into daily aims.
- Act happy. Put on a happy face; carry smiling

expressions. Talk as if you feel positive.
- Seek work and leisure that engages your skills. Happy people often are in a zone called "flow" - absorbed in a task that challenges them without overwhelming them.
- Exercise. Aerobic exercise not only promises health and energy, it is an antidote to mild depression.
- Give your body the sleep it wants.
- Give priority to close relationship.
- Focus beyond the self. Reach out to those in need.
- Keep a gratitude journal. On daily basis, keep a record of giving and receiving the good.
- Nurture your spiritual self.

Building Flourishing Relationship

The capacity for love is a central component of all human societies. Love in all its manifestations, whether for children, parents, friends, or romantic partners, gives depth to human relationships. Specifically, love brings people close to each other physically and emotionally. When experienced intensely, it makes people feel expansively about themselves and the world.

While love has been depicted in classical literature in the past, contemporary behavioural scientists have attempted to identify its various components at an empirical level. Love for a companion is considered central to life well lived. Romantic love may not be essential in life, but it may be essential for joy. Life without love would be for many people like a black-and-white movie full of events and activities but without the colour that gives vibrancy and provides a sense of celebration.

A step-wise conceptualization of romantic love may foster an understanding of how it develops between two people.

Stage 1: Passionate and Companionate Aspects.

Romantic love is a complex emotion that may be best parsed into *passionate* and *companionate* forms. Passionate love (the intense arousal that fuels a romantic union) involves a state of absorption between two people that often is accompanied by moods ranging from ecstasy to anguish. Companionate love (the soothing, steady warmth that sustains a relationship) is manifested on a strong bond and intertwining of lives that bring about feelings of comfort and peace. These two forms can occur simultaneously or intermittently rather than sequentially.

Romantic love is characterized by intense arousal and warm affection. During these stage partners seek knowledge about each other, they also use this knowledge to further their relationship. In a study of college students who were probably in the early stages of romantic relationship, nearly half named their romantic partners when asked to identify their closest friend. This suggests that passionate and companionate love can coexist in the new relationships of young people. Likewise in a study of couples married for as long as 40 years, researchers found that companionate love and passionate love were alive, and that passionate love was the strongest predictor of marital satisfaction.

Stage 2: The Triangular Components of Love.

In developing a triangular theory of love, psychologist Robert Sternberg opine that love is a mix of three components: (1) passion, or physical attractiveness and romantic drives, (2) intimacy, or feeling of closeness and connectedness, and (3) commitment, involving the decision to initiate and sustain a relationship. Various combinations of these three components held eight forms of love. For example, intimacy and passion combined produce romantic love, whereas intimacy and commitment together constitute companionate love. Consummate love, the most durable type, is manifested when all three components (passion, intimacy and commitment) are present at high levels and in balance across both partners.

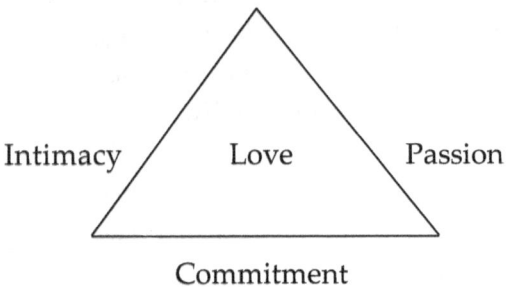

Consummate (Couple) Love = Intimacy + Commitment + Passion
Romantic Love = Intimacy + Passion
Friendship = Intimacy + Commitment
Infatuation = Passion only
Empty Love = Commitment only
(Commercial Relation)
Fatuous Love = Passion + Commitment

Intimacy refers to mutual understanding, warm affection and mutual concern for the other's welfare. **Passion** means strong emotion, excitement, and physical arousal, often tied to sexual desire and attraction. **Commitment** is the conscious decision to stay in a relationship for a long period. It includes a series of devotion to the relationship and a willingness, to work on maintaining it. By putting together different combinations of the three ingredients, Sternberg's model describes several varieties of love and the specific components of romantic and companionate love.

High intimacy and passion describes romantic love in Sternberg's model. It may seem strange not to include commitment, but Sternberg argues that commitment is not a defining feature of romantic love. A winter romance, for example, may involve intimate mutual disclosure and strong passion, but no commitment to continue the relationship at winter's end.

Companionate love is a slow-developing love built on high intimacy and strong commitment. When youthful passion fades in a marriage, companionate love, based on deep, affectionate friendship provides a solid foundation for a lasting and successful relationship.

Both **fatuous love** (passion + commitment) and **infatuated love** (passion only) types might be regarded as forms of immature, blind or unreasonable love built on passion. Fatuous love combines high passion and commitment with an absence of intimacy. This would describe people who hardly know each other, but are caught up in a whirlwind passionate romance. Their commitment is based on passion and sustained solely by passion. Because passion is likely to fade with time, fatuous love relationships are unlikely to last. The same can be said for infatuated love, based only on passion, without intimacy or commitment. This might describe a teen romance in which sexual passion is taken for love. Infatuated love may also describe the sense of awe, adoration, and sex-related feelings that some people have for their favorite. Bollywood movie or music celebrity.

Empty Love (commitment only) includes no passion, no intimacy, just a commitment to stay together. Appropriately called empty love, this would describe an emotionally "dead" relationship that both members find some reason to continue. Reasons might include things such as convenience financial benefits, a sense of obligation or duty.

Consummate or complete love (intimacy + passion + commitment) is marked by high intimacy, passion and commitment. It is a form of love that many people desire. As in romantic love, the passionate component typically decreases over time. Yet, other components remain strong and grow. Sternberg's three-component model of love has received good empirical support. People's understanding of love's primary features and the differences among various types of relationships appear to fit well with the intimacy / passion / commitment conception. It is obvious to surmise that these components grow as love becomes more and more mature and sustainable.

Stage 3: The Self-Expansion of Romantic Love

Humans have a basic motivation to expand the self; the emotions, cognitions and behaviours of love fuel such self-expansion. People seek to expand themselves through love.

According to self-expansion theory, relationship satisfaction is a natural by-product of self-expressive love. Being in a loving relationship makes people feel good. They then associate these positive feelings with the relationship, thereby reinforcing their commitment to relationship. The positive consequences of being in love are clear. Researchers find that those who fall in love experience increased self-esteem and self-efficacy. On a more cognitive level, self-expansion means that each partner has made a decision to include another in his or her self. This investment in each other adds to relationship satisfaction. Each of the partners makes a greater use of the expression "we" instead of "I".

This inclusively is a prominent feature of flourishing relationship.

Another relationship involves a culture of appreciation. Generally it is a human weakness that we tend to explain our success in terms of internal (dispositional) factors and explain failure in terms of external (environmental) factors. For example, we consider ourselves as bright if we complete a work successfully. In contrast, we blame the situational (environmental) difficulty if we fail. But we do not use similar yard sticks to explain others' success / failure. If others succeed, we give credit to situational parameters. If others fail, we blame their dispositional (personality) inadequacy.

What about the explanatory style in the context of flourishing relationship? If a wife fails in fixing the dinner in time, how does the husband explain the event? Is it because of the carelessness of wife or because of some unexpected arrival of guests in home? Needless to say as relationship flourishes, each of the partners takes an adaptive explanatory style. For success, he/she appreciates the other's positive disposition. For failure, he/she looks at the environmental constraints. This kind of explanatory style is a mark of maturing relationship.

The research on love also describes the meaning of "I love you". In a number of studies, the meaning of the statement, "I love you" has been analyzed. When participants are asked to describe exactly what they meant when they say "I love you" a variety of answers are generated. Some of the answers include: I understand; I support you, I am thankful to you. Ours is a good life; It is good to be with you. The variability in the meaning of these expressions suggests the complexity and richness of the emotion of love.

Well-minded relationships are healthy and long lasting. The following exhibit depicts the sequence in flourishing relationship.

Adaptive	Nonadaptive
• An in-depth knowing process both partners seek to know and to be known by the other	No special effort to know or to be known by other
• Both partners use the knowledge gained in enhancing relationship	Knowledge gained is not used
• Both partners accept what they learn and respect the other for the person they learn about	Acceptance of what is learned is low
• Both partners in time develop a sense of being special and appreciated in the relationship	One or both partners fail to develop a sense of being special and appreciated in the relationship

Positive Life Events

Stressful life events are a familiar and much studied source of unhappiness, mental and physical ill-health. **Positive Life Events (PLE)** have similar effects in opposite direction. The kind of positive events we have in mind are sports and exercise, social events, success, recognition at work and meetings of leisure groups. Some PLEs are accidental, such as gifts, invitations, unexpected meetings, success, and falling in love. Yet a number of PLEs can be sought such as watching a fascinating movie. Seeking PLEs and making them a part of personal life may be very helpful in mood induction procedure.

While PLEs are culture-linked, broad categories of PLEs can be presented.

- **Social events**. There are many kinds of these. Being in love is a source of intense joy and increased self-esteem, being with friends produce companionship and positive feelings. Sometimes company of family members affords pleasure.
- **Sport and exercise.** Produce positive moods and greater happiness when done regularly, and the effect may last to the next day. The quality of experience is of increased arousal, and self-esteem, as well enjoyment of the social relations involved.
- **Religion and music** are quite intense for those

involved, including other worldly feelings of loss of sense of self, timelessness, glimpsing another world.
- **Leisure groups** of other kinds are a source of PLEs, sometimes several aspects of experience combine, such as dancing which involves music, exercise and social interaction.
- **Work.** Positive experience here are mainly reported for success and recognition, through job satisfaction studies find that intrinsic satisfaction comes from use of skills and social satisfaction from relations with workmates.
- **Watching TV** is a great enigma. It is done so much that it must be rewarding, but research finds that it produces only weak positive moods, and watchers are often half-asleep. However, moods it produces are positive.
- **Holidays,** though not frequent, can be looked forward to, and are great source of relaxation, adventure and pleasure.

Different sections of the community have different frequencies of events; working-class people have more of those linked with poverty, unemployment and affordability. Similar students' populations tend to prefer some specific PLEs. The listings below indicate weightages (out of 100 units) of different PLEs as shown by Oxford students.

Events	Weightages
Falling in love	78.1
Passing an exam (gaining a certificate)	75.5
Recovering from a serious illness	72.1
Making it up after an argument	66.0
Getting married or engaged	65.0
Birth of a child	64.6
Wining a lot of money	64.4
Getting promoted at work	59.9

    Going out with friends   58.0
    Getting a new job   56.1

PLEs are good for physical and psychological health. Increasing PLEs is a successful way of enhancing happiness and reducing anxiety and depression.

Spirituality

Spirituality as a topic in psychology has received mixed receptions. A number of psychologists in the 20th century ignored it; some psychologists viewed this as a topic in philosophy while others equated it with psychopathology. Despite such neglect, spirituality can't be dismissed as a "cultural fact". A vast majority of people believe in God and believe that God can be reached through prayer. People also believe that religion is important or very important in their lives. The importance of spirituality is perceived in a number of domains of human functioning such as mental health use of drug and alcohol, parenting, marital functioning and morality.

Defining Spirituality

Although many people describe themselves as spiritual, they define the term in many different ways. Definitions of spirituality have ranged from the best of that which is human to a quest for existential meaning, to the transcendent human dimension.

Traditionally many people equate spirituality with religious behaviour. However, contemporary writes contrast the two, suggesting that religion is dogmatic, institutional, and restrictive, whereas spirituality is personal, subjective and life-enhancing. Spirituality represents the key and unique function of religion. Spirituality is defined as **"a search for the sacred"**.

There are two key terms in this definition: search and the sacred. The term search indicates that spirituality is a process, one that involves efforts to discover the sacred and one that involves efforts to hold onto the sacred once it has been found. People can take a virtually limitless number of pathways in their attempts to discover and conserve the sacred. Spiritual pathways include social involvements that range from traditional religious institutions to non-traditional spiritual groups, programs and associations (e.g. Twelve Step meditation centers, Scientology). Pathways involve systems of belief that include those of traditional organized religions (Hindu, etc), newer spirituality movements (e.g. feminist, godless, ecological spiritualities), and more individualized world views.

In the *Oxford English Dictionary*, the word *sacred* is defined as the holy. The sacred includes concept of God, the divine and the transcendent. However, other objects can become sacred or take on an extra-ordinary power by virtue of their association with, or representations of divinity. Sacred objects include time and space (temples), events and transitions (birth and death), materials (cross), cultural products (music, literature), people (saints), social attributes (compassion), psychological attributes (meaning). We would describe persons to be spiritual to the extent they are trying to find, know, experience, or relate to what they perceive as sacred.

The Discovery of the Scared

The search for God begins in childhood. Some scientists have suggested that there is an *innate genetic* basis for spirituality. Others have emphasized that conceptions of God are rooted in the child's intrapsychic capacity to symbolize, fantasize and create superhuman beings. Some have asserted that spirituality grows out of critical life events and challenges that reveal human limitations. And others have emphasized the importance of the social context (familial, institutional, cultural) in shaping the child's understanding of God.

Empirical research on the origins of spirituality is not plentiful. Kirkpatrik suggests that child's mental models of God are likely to correspond to the models of self and others that emerge out of repeat interactions with primary attachment figures (e.g. mother or father)

The Conservation of the Sacred

The search does not end after the sacred has been discovered. Once found, people strive to hold on to the sacred.

There are a number of spiritual methods for conserving the individual's relationship with the sacred. People sustain their relationship by prayer, meditation, and experiencing the spiritual dimension in daily life.

Spirituality offers a unique set of resources for living. Social scientists, health professionals and mental health professionals are striving to develop psychospiritual interventions that integrate spiritual resources into clinical practice.

The Buffering Role of Humour

Humour is a topic of central concern in psychology and philosophy. It is observed that on an average, children laugh 300 times a day and adults only laugh five times a day. Since children laugh more than adults, it seems that our sense of humour dwindles as we become more aware and educated of the world. Without any central definition of humour utilized in the world of psychology, University of Western Ontario professor, Rod Martin, was prompted to write a unifying book that investigated the role of humour. He defined it as: "**A process (that) can be divided into four essential components: (a) a social context, (b) a cognitive-perceptual process, (c) an emotional response, and (d) the vocal-behavioural expression of laughter."**

Theories of Humour

A number of theories have been advanced in the context of humour.

Humour congruity theory. The Incongruity Theory says that humour is the perception of something incongruous – something that violates our mental patterns and expectations. In simple terms people laugh at things that surprise them because of the context in which it is presented: things are incongruent (out of place) within the context of which they are delivered.

One way to further explain the theory, humorous amusement is not just any response to incongruity but a way of enjoying incongruity. The following three features may be noted:

1. A person perceives (thinks, imagines) an object as being incongruous.
2. The person enjoys perceiving (thinking, imagining) the object
3. The person enjoys the perceived (thought, imagined) incongruity at least partly for itself, rather than solely for some ulterior reason.

This approach to joking is similar to techniques of stand-up and the punch (line). The set-up is the first part of the joke: it creates the expectation. The punch (line) is the last part that violates that expectation. In the language of the incongruity theory, the joke's ending is incongruous with the beginning.

Humour superiority theory. The theory suggests that when people make a stupid mistake, are the victim of an unfortunate situation, or misunderstand an obvious instruction, they look stupid in a social environment. Thus, we laugh at these jokes, people, and situations because it makes us feel superior to the victim and their unfortunate luck.

Simply put, our laughter expresses feelings of superiority over other people or over a former state of ourselves. However, some critics argued that the feeling of superiority is neither necessary nor sufficient for laughter. Sometimes we laugh when a comic character shows surprising skill that we lack. Some people too, laugh at themselves – not a former state of themselves, but what is happening now. Cases of pity are also cited. A gentleman riding a coach who sees ragged beggars on the street for example, will feel that he is better off than they, but such feelings are unlikely to amuse him. In such cases we are in greater danger of weeping than laughing.

Tension release theory. According to Freud, jokes and laughter are a way in which people could release their sexual or aggressive thoughts in a socially acceptable way. Freud proposed that it served as a way to cope with the problems and issues in our lives that we are hesitant to confront in another way, thus it provides a source of relief to these thoughts unconsciously. By attempting to cope with varying emotions and thoughts, laughter is a way to release the tension that was built.

The release, Freud said, would be triggered by the dramatic or surprising occurrence in the punchline. But many dramatic surprises are not pleasant at all, and jokes that are neither aggressive nor sexual can work on us regardless of how tense we are.

Humour benign violation theory. This theory holds that humour occurs when three specific conditions are satisfied
a) a situation is a violation
b) the situation is benign
c) both perceptions occur simultaneously

The violations are strictly based on how an individual believes the world should be. This theory is important because it accounts for the thresholds of what is and what is not funny. It explains that a situation may not be funny because the violation isn't simultaneously benign, or because it is beginning without a social violation.

Humour Styles

Over a decade ago, Rod Martin and his colleagues (2003) developed a model of humour styles that has since become one of the main theoretical frameworks used to guide psychological research on sense of humour. It describes four distinct styles of humour on the basis of whether it enhances self or relationship with others combined with the effect it has, be it injurious or benign. These styles have differential impact on psychological well-being and psychological functioning.

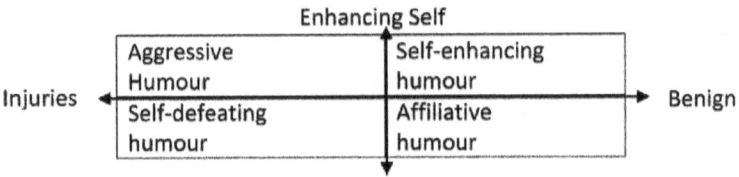

Affiliative humour. Individuals high in this dimension often use humour as a way to charm and amuse others, ease tension among others, and improve relationships. The goal is to create a sense of fellowship, happiness and well-being.

Individuals who report high levels of affiliative humour are more likely to initiate friendship. In an organizational setting, affiliate humour has been shown to increase group cohesiveness and promote creativity in the workplace. It is also associated with increased levels of self-esteem, well-being, emotional stability, and social intimacy. This style of humour is linked with decreased levels of depression and anxiety.

Aggressive humour. It is a style of humour that is potentially detrimental towards others. This involves put-downs, insults, criticism or sarcasm targeted towards individuals. Prejudices such as racism and sexism are considered to be the aggressive styles of humour. This type of humour may at times seem like playful fun, but sometimes the underlying intent is to harm or belittle others.

Self-enhancing humour. This is being able to laugh at yourself, such as making a joke when something bad has happened to you in constructive, non-detrimental manner trying to find the humour in everyday situations and making yourself the target of the humour in a good-natured way. It is related to healthy coping with stress. It is emotion-regulating humour in which individuals use humour to look on the bright side of a bad situation, find the silver lining or maintain a positive attitude even in trying times.

Self-defeating humour. It is the style of humour characterized by the use of potentially detrimental humour towards the self in order to gain approval from others. Psychologically, this can be an unhealthy form of humour. It is sometimes used by targets of bullies to try to avoid attacks – making oneself the buff of jokes before others put you down. Individuals who use this type of humour tend to have higher levels of neuroticism and lower levels of agreeableness and conscientiousness. Self-defeating humour is also associated with higher levels of anxiety, depression and psychiatric symptoms. It is also linked with lower levels of self-esteem, well-being and intimacy.

Considerable research has documented that the increased use of self-enhancing and affiliative humour can facilitate psychological well-being and enhance interpersonal relationships, whereas greater use of self-defeating and aggressive humour can be detrimental.

Humour in Daily Lives

Humour as a defense mechanism: A common response that serves as a defense mechanism. In serious situations humour is an attempt to protect the person from having to face an uncomfortable situation.

- Buffering effect on stress: Stressful experiences,

especially those of a chronic nature, may contribute towards a variety of adverse health outcomes. A bulk of research has shown that humour could be a coping mechanism or moderator that lessons the impact of frequent stressors.

- Benefits of humour in workplace: Humour promotes both productivity and creativity in workplace. Companies such as Zappos and Southwest Airlines have used humour and a positive fun culture to help brand their business, attract and retain employees and to attract customers.

Positive Moods and Immune Functioning

It is a common observation that a number of students catch cold during their examination period. Psychological stress seems able to alter susceptibility to infectious agents, influencing the onset course and outcome of certain infectious pathologies. When demands imposed by events exceed individual's abilities to cope, a psychological stress response composed of negative cognitive and emotional states is elicited. It is these responses that are thought to influence immune function through their effects on behavior coping and neuroendocrine responses.

These two statements exemplify, what research in psychoneuroimmunology has demonstrated. **Psychoneuroimmunology (PNI)** explains interrelationships among psychological processes and neurons, endocrine and immune system functioning. Tremendous advances have been made in our understanding of the role the psychology plays in the stability of the human immune system. Much PNI research has stressed on the impact that physical stress or emotions have on immune functioning.

The immune system in the body is a means of guarding against foreign invaders such as bacteria, viruses and carcinogenic substances. Immune system protection is of two types: *nonspecific immunity* and *specific immunity*. The first involves several mechanisms: actual barriers (such as the skin, which can keep out invaders), phagocytosis (the process whereby special white blood cells engulf and destroy pathogens), inflammation (swelling and increased blood flow that facilitates the movement and function of white blood cells), and the secretion of toxic chemicals (to destroy microorganisms such as bacteria and viruses). The second type specific immunity involves the body's ability to protect itself from specific invaders. An example would be the immune response to an encounter with the measles virus after antibodies have been developed from immunization.

There are two kinds of specific immunological reactions: *humoral immunity* and *cell-mediated immunity*. Humoral immunity occurs when an antigen (a threatening agent) stimulates B lymphocytes to differentiate into cells that secrete antibodies to fight a foreign invader. Cell-mediated immunity on the other hand, involves T-lymphocytes from the thymes gland and is slower acting. A T-cell is a type of infection fighting white blood cell. T-cell levels and lymphocyte activity are key elements in immune functioning. Instead of releasing anti-bodies into the blood, cell-medicated immunity occurs in the following way. When stimulated by an antigen, T-cells secrete chemicals that aid in a process by which attacking microorganisms are ingested and destroyed. Some T-cells (called helper T-cells) appear to aid to humoral immunity, whereas suppressor T-cells may suppress humoral reactions. Many other cells and components of the blood are also involved in immune responses: most cells, monocytes macrophages, natural killer (NK) cells, and several others.

The activity of natural killer (NK) cells in immune

response to stress illustrates the complexity of immune system responses. First, the effects of acute stress on NK cells have been shown to be both positive and negative, depending upon certain factors. One determinant is the time at which NK activity is measured following an acute stressor. NK activity tends to be increased during or immediately after a stressful activity, whereas NK activity tends to decrease later (such as 48 or 72 hours following an stressor). The age of the individuals under study also matters. In younger women (ages 21-41), NK activity was increased following a 12-minute stressful arithmetic task, but no such increased activity was seen for older women.

Mood and Immune Functioning

Research evidence supports the idea that physical symptoms are related to mental status. PNI research has found that individuals under severe, chronic stress are more likely to develop symptoms from exposure to the rhinovirus (the common cold) than are individuals under no or only acute stress. Individuals reporting greater levels of positive mood over a two-day period have higher levels of natural killer cell activity (a measure of immune functioning) than do those reporting negative moods over the same two days. Antibody levels have been found among men to be higher on those days in which they reported a positive mood. Furthermore, individuals exposed to a humorous film showed higher levels of salivary immunoglobulin-A (a measure of immune functioning) than did those exposed to a non-humorous comparison film. Another study found that while medical students were undergoing the stress of exams, their levels of salivary IgA were suppressed far more than six days following the examination period. Those with suppressed immune functioning did not necessarily acquire an upper respiratory tract infection, however. Perhaps it was the youth and general good health of those students that allowed them to avoid catching a cold despite their suppressed immune system, or perhaps they were lucky enough to have not been exposed to the cold virus.

In another study a small group of patients who suffered from recurrent oral herps (cold sore) was followed over three months and provided ratings of their stress and daily mood fluctuations. Findings showed that cold-sore outbreaks did vary with stress and mood fluctuations, indicating that the immune system was suppressed enough during stress to allow for the manifestation. In fact, the week before the outbreak there was a significant reduction in subjects' level of natural killer cells in their blood. Another interesting and innovative study examined speed with which the body heals under varying levels of stress. Dental students were given two small wounds in their hard palates, one during the summer vacation and one right before exams. Wounds healed 40 percent slower just prior to exams, which can reasonably be assumed to be a time of higher stress.

PNI research supports that as stress increases, the nervous system responds by increasing cortisol levels, blood pressure, and epinephrine. In turn these act to suppress immune functioning. Stress also works directly on IgA, another indicator of immune functioning. What must be remembered, however is that interaction of the immune system with other systems (physical and mental) are extremely complex. For example, numerous studies have found significant beneficial effects of social support on the immune functioning.

Skills to Manage Fear in an Unsafe World

The recent out-break of Corona in China and its spread to almost all countries of world has generated a climate of fear and anxiety. The panic situations both in the developed as well as developing countries have created phobic reactions on the part of the entire world. Although all countries of the world are taking nation-wise and world-wide steps to prevent its spread, the external arrangements do not seem to be adequate. It appears that a special form of **psychological resilience** is needed to get around the problem of corona virus threat.

Below are some things people can do to help themselves cope with this threatening situation. It is important to spend time and energy strengthening our internal resources, so we can feel more competent in deal with this difficult event.

1. **Accept Your Feeling**
   Realize that events of this magnitude take time to process. Even if you are not directly affected, exposure to constant media coverage can be traumatizing. Give yourself time to feel sad or introspective. These are normal human reactions.

2. **Re-establish Your Usual Routines**
    Don't spend all day watching news coverage. Sleep, exercise, healthy eating, pleasant activities, time with friends and family, yoga or mediation can strengthen your internal resources to cope.
3. **Create a Mental Safe Place**
    Mentally create a peaceful and relaxing setting in your mind to help you de-stress. Deliberately focus on each sense at a time. What do you see, hear, smell, and feel in the real or imaginary heaven and peace?
4. **Find Self-Compassion**
    Treat yourself and your feeling with tenderness and compassion. Do not push feelings away. Rather find or create a soothing environment in which to feel them. This may be with a friend or family member, while listening to soothing music. Mindful meditation, with its dual focus on observing the breath and letting sensations come up, provides an excellent way of looking at feelings while remaining anchored in the present.
5. **Create a Narrative**
    Write a narrative of how you found about the event, the details that upset you, and your thoughts and feelings. Writing helps you to organize your reactions into a narrative that makes your reactions clearer and more understandable. "When we name it, we can tame it".
6. **Seek Support and Connection**
    Reach out to others who can provide support and comfort. If you need to talk about your feelings, choose a person who can listen and be with you as you struggle with anxiety. Stay away from people who minimize your feeling and tell you to "Get over

it". Social support is one of the most important predictors of fear-reduction.

7. **Turn to the Positive**
Remind yourself that although the world contains much suffering, it also contains much that is good. Deliberately think about the positive and uplifting things in your own life and community. Think about the freedom and opportunities you have that many in the world have not. Focus on the strengths and coping strategies you have developed and the people you can turn to for help if you need it.

8. **Recommit to Your Most Important Values**
Think about your most important personal or spiritual values, including love for family, nonviolence, compassion, integrity, hard work, and so on. How does your current life reflect these values? Make a list of your values and some concrete steps you can take in the next week or month to make them an important part of your life.

9. **Feel Gratitude**
Focus on the people of your life, past and present, that have provided you with protection, nurturance, or love. Bring to mind an image of yourself with that person. Focus on how you feel in that person's presence. Think about the gratitude you feel for what that person has given you. Find a concrete way to express that gratitude, through demonstration of affection, a letter, a gift, or just telling them you appreciate them.

10. **Do Something Constructive**
Chanel your fear and anxiety into constructive activities to help improve the situation. This may include sending letters of support to the victims

volunteering at shelters, writing letters to the editors of local papers. Taking action can combat feelings of helplessness or guilt and can contribute to increasing goodness in the world.

Additional Steps

1. **Take time out**

    It feels impossible to think clearly when you are flooded with fear or anxiety. A racing heart, sweating palms and feeling panicky and confused are the result of adrenalin (a stress hormone). So the first thing to do is to take time so that you can physically calm down. Distract yourself from the worry for 15 minutes by walking around the block, making a cup of tea, or having a bath. When you're physically calmed down, you'll feel better able to decide on the best way to cope.

2. **What's the worst that can happen?**

    When you are anxious about something it can help you to think through what the worst end result could be. Sometimes the worst that can happen is a panic attack. If you start to get a faster heartbeat or sweating palms the best thing is not to fight it. Stay where you are and simply feel the panic without trying to distract yourself. Placing the palm of your hand on your stomach and breathing slowly and deeply (no more than 12 breaths a minute) helps soothe the body. It may take up to an hour, but eventually the panic will go away on its own. The goal is to help the mind get used to coping with panic, which takes the fear of fear away.

3. **Expose yourself to the fear**

    Avoiding fears only make them scarier. If you panic

one day getting into a lift, it's best to get back into a lift the next day. Stand in the lift and feel the fear until it goes away. Whatever your fear, if you face it, it should start to fade.

4. **Welcome the worst**
   Each time fear is embraced, it makes them easier to cope with the next time they strike, until in the end they are no longer a problem. Try imagining the worst thing that can happen – perhaps it's panicking and having a heart attack. Then try to think yourself into having a heart attack. It's just not possible. The fear will run away the more you chase it.

5. **Get real**
   Fears tend to be much worse than reality. Often, people who have been victims can't help thinking they are going to be victims again. But the chances that this will happen again is actually very low.

6. **Don't expect perfection**
   Life is full of stresses. Yet many of us feel that our lives must be perfect. Bad days and setback will always happen, and it is essential to remember that life is messy.

7. **Visualize**
   Take a moment to close your eyes and imagine a place of safety and calm – it could be a picture of you walking on a beautiful beach or happy memory from childhood. Let the positive feeling soothe you until you feel more relaxed.

8. **Talk about it**
   Sharing fears takes a lot of their scariness. If you can't talk to a partner, friend or family member, call someone you love.

9. **Go back to basics**

A good sleep, a wholesome meal and a walk are often the best cures for anxiety. The easiest way to fall asleep when worries are spiraling through the mind can be to stop trying to sleep, instead try to stay awake.

Many people turn to alcohol or drugs to self-treat anxiety with the idea that it will make them feel better, but these only make nervousness worse. On the other hand, eating well will make your feel better.

10. **Reward yourself**

Finally give yourself a treat. Reinforce yourself by some activity such as taking a country walk, dining out, reading a book or whatever little gift makes you happy.

How to Control Your Anger

Anger is an emotional state that varies from minor irritation to intense fury. Like other emotions, it is accompanied by physiological and biological changes. When you get angry, your heart rate and blood pressure go up, as do the levels of your energy hormones, adrenaline and noradrenaline. Anger can be caused by both external and internal events. You could be angry at a specific person (your colleagues or boss), or an event (such as traffic jam), or your anger could be caused by worrying about your personal problems.

The instinctive natural way to express anger is to respond aggressively. Anger is a natural adaptive response to threats. It inspires powerful, often aggressive, feeling and behaviours which allow us to fight and to defend ourselves when we are attacked. A certain amount of anger, therefore, is necessary to our survival.

On the other hand, we can't physically lash out at every person or object that irritates or annoys us. People use a variety of both conscious and unconscious processes to deal with their angry feelings. The three main approaches are expressing, suppressing and calming. Expressing your angry feeling in an assertive – not aggressive – manner is the healthiest way to express anger. To do this, you have to learn how to make clear what your needs are, and how to get them met, without hurting others. Being assertive does not mean being pushy or demanding. It means being respectful of yourself. Anger can be suppressed and then converted or redirected. This happens when you hold in your anger, stop thinking about it and focus on something positive. The aim is to inhibit or suppress your anger and convert it into more constructive behaviour. The danger in this type of response is that if it isn't allowed outward expression, your anger can turn inward – on yourself. Anger turned inward may cause hypertension, high blood pressure, or depression. Unexpressed anger can create other problems. Finally, you can calm down inside. This means not just controlling your outward behaviour but also controlling your internal responses, taking steps to lower your heart rate, calm yourself down, and let the feeling subside.

Some people believe that it is good to let all anger out. This is a dangerous myth. Research has found that "letting it rip" with anger actually escalates anger and aggression and does nothing to help you resolve the situation. It is best to find out what it is that triggers your anger, and then to develop strategies to keep those triggers from tipping you over that edge.

Strategies to Keep Anger at Bay
A number of strategies are listed below:
    Relaxation. Simple relaxation tools, such as deep breathing and relaxing imagery, can help calm down angry feelings. There are books and courses that can teach you relaxation techniques, and once you learn the techniques, you can call upon them in any situation.
Some sample steps you can try:
- Breathe deeply, from your diaphragm, breathing from

your chest won't relax you. Picture your breath coming up from your "gut".
- Slowly repeat a calm word or phrase such as "relax", "take it easy". Repeat it to yourself while breathing deeply.
- Use imagery, visualize a relaxing experience, from either your memory or your imagination.
- Nonstrenuous, slow yoga-like exercise can relax your muscles and make you feel much calmer.
- Practice these techniques daily. Learn to use them automatically when you are in a tense situation.

Cognitive restructuring. Many people get into anger because of their faulty thoughts. They use extreme words in their thoughts and expressions. They use words like "never" or "always". In order to reduce and eliminate anger, they need to replace their faulty thoughts by more rational thinking. Remind yourself that getting angry is not going to fix anything. Reality appraisals would eliminate a significant portion of your anger.

Problem solving. Sometimes, our anger and frustrations are caused by very real and inescapable problems in our lives. Yet every problem has a solution. Instead of dwelling on the problem, it is better to analyze the problem and plan solution. Do not fall into all-or-nothing thinking, even if the problem does not get solved right away.

Better communication. Angry people tend to jump to — and act on – conclusions, and some of those conclusions can be very inaccurate. The first thing is to slow down and think judiciously. Don't say the first thing that comes to your head, but slow down and think carefully about what you went to say. At the same time, listen carefully to what the other person is saying and take your time before answering.

Use humour. Humour can help defuse rage in a number of ways. For one thing it can help you get a more balanced perspective. When you get angry and call someone a name or refer to them in some imaginative phrase stop and picture what that word would literally look like. If you are at work and you think of a coworker as a "dirtbag", for example, picture a large bag full of dirt, sitting at your colleague's desk, talking on the phone, going to meetings. Do those whenever a name comes to your head about another person. If you can draw a picture of what the actual thing might look like. This will take a lot of the edge off your fury, and humour can always be relied on to help unknot a tense situation.

Changing your environment. Sometimes it's our immediate surroundings that give us cause for irritation and fury. Problems and responsibilities can weigh on you and make you feel angry at the "trap" you seem to have fallen into and all the people and things that form that trap. Give yourself a break. Make sure you have some "personal time" scheduled for times of the day that you know are particularly stressful. One example is the working mothers who has a standing rule that when she comes home from work for the first 15 minutes "nobody talks to Mom unless the house in on fire". After this brief quiet time, she feels better prepared to handle demands from her kids without blowing up at them.

Some other tips. If your child's chaotic room makes you furious every time you walk by it, shut the door. Don't make yourself look at what infuriates you. Avoidance: Find alternatives. If your daily commute through traffic leaves you in a state of rage, map out a different route, one that's less congested or more scenic. Or find another alternative, such as a bus or commuter train.

Need for counselling. If you feel that your anger is really out of control, if it is having an impact on your relationships and on important parts of your life, you might consider counselling to learn how to handle it better. A psychologist or other licensed mental health professional can work with you in developing a range of techniques for changing your thinking and your behaviour.

Meditation

Meditation actually comprises a family of techniques that go by different names (Zen meditation, Transcendental Meditation, Vipassana meditation) and different categories (concentrative mindfulness, contemplative loving-kindness). The core element that underlies all of them is the cultivation of attention. Of course, you can focus attention in many different ways – for example, nonanalytically and nonemotionally on a single object (on a flame, your breath, a sound, or a single word, such as is done in concentrative meditation, or nonjudgmentally on all thoughts, sights, and sounds without ruminating on them (such as is done in mindfulness meditation), or more broadly by opening yourself to God to contemplate the big questions of life (such as is done in contemplative mediation). Meditation is a personal experience and may be performed in many different ways. Yet certain core elements are recognized:

- Be nonjudgmental. Observe the present moment impartially, with detachment, without evaluation.
- Be nonstriving. Although you are a person committed to goals, don't struggle mentally while meditating.
- Be patient. Don't rush or force things but allow them to unfold in their own good time.

- Be trusting. Trust yourself and trust that things will work out in life.
- Be open. Pay attention to every little thing, as though you were seeing it for the very first time.
- Let go. Set yourself free of rumination. This is what is called nonattachment.

The Process

Researchers who study the bodies of people during the practice of meditation have confirmed that mediators are able to attain a profound state of physiological rest (indicated by a reduced respiration rate, for instance) and a heightened state of awareness and alertness (indicated by such things as increased blood flow and other relevant markers in the brain). Lyubomirsky (2007) conducted a study in which healthy workers underwent an eight-week training practice in mindfulness meditation. At the end of the eight week those who practiced meditation (compared with a control group) showed increases in their left-frontal cortex, relative to the right. It may be indicated that this particular pattern of greater brain activity in the left versus right part of the brain is observed in happy and approach-oriented individuals. This supports other studies indicating greater happiness and lower depression and anxiety in meditators.

Not surprisingly such physiological effects may translate into and influence a person's health. Meditation interventions have been shown to be effective in patients with heart diseases, chronic pain, skin disorders and a variety of mental health conditions such as depression, anxiety, panic, and substance abuse. Besides these direct benefits, meditation reduces reactivity to stress and boosts self-esteem, positive moods and feelings of control.

A number of intriguing studies have even revealed benefits of meditation for such seemingly intractable characteristics as intelligence, creativity and cognitive flexibility in the elderly.

The Technique

Teachers of meditation advise that mediating involves sitting alone in a comfortable place, back straight. Close your eyes and focus on breathing in and out. As you breathe out, silently repeat a short word (like *one, aum,* or *be*). Or if you prefer, focus on a specific object, sound, or task, like a candle, a tone, or your breath. If your mind wanders (e.g. I have to take my lunch), let your thoughts pass, and then restart by bringing your attention back to your breath. The key is to notice your mind wandering and then to turn inward and "detach" from your thought. Don't let your ruminations and fantasies and plans and memories control you, take charge of them. This will take practice and repetition, beginners usually can only "quiet" or "still" the mind for no more than a few seconds at a time. A common experience is that the moment you think you've emptied your mind, it starts to fill up again.

Build the length of time you are able to meditate from five to twenty minutes and try to do it every day. Ideally arrange for a meditation space. It can be modest or large, decorated – with photos, artworks, or inspirational contents. It should be comfortable and, if possible, free of disattractions.

Meditation has many regards, but it does not come effortlessly Pascal commented" "All of humanity's problems seem from man's inability to sit quietly in a room alone".

Building Psychological Resilience

Exceptional events trigger exceptional insights. It is a common observation that great discoveries and inventions are not limited to laboratories. Sometimes extraordinary events taking place in societies, unique happenings in human lives and unusual circumstances occurring in the globe engage our attention. Many people are elated or frightened; yet a few of us pursue certain interesting aspect of the event and come across a wonderful law of universal significance. The concept of psychological resilience is one such unique law.

In 1945, following World War II an orphanage in the village of Lingfield in Surrey, England, arranged to take twenty-four young child survivors of the Holocaust. Most of the children, between the ages of three and eight years old were either arriving from concentration camps like Auschwitz and Terezin or had been living in hiding. They were already victims of traumatic stress. Children from the Terezin group had been present at mass hanging and many of them had been forced to pass boxes of human ashes back and forth. The Auschwitz children had been surrounded by the stench of dead bodies, waking to the sight of the crematoria smoke each day.

The four youngest children were only months old when they arrived in the Terezin concentration camp.

Subsequently they were placed in the Lingfield orphanage. In 1979, when all four of them were thirty-seven, an American psychologist named Sarah Moscovitz found these child survivors (originally described by Anna Freud, Sigmund Freud's daughter). She conducted a series of interviews with them both in 1979 and 1984, to document their progress over time.

Berl and Leah, the smallest and the weakest of the youngest four, suffered the most. They struggled socially and academically. They survived but they struggled, riddled with anxiety, shame and sadness about the past. More surprising were the interviews with Jack and Bella, the other two members. When Moscovitz met him, Jack was happily married with a supportive wife and two children. He owned his taxi in London and he described his pleasure of meeting new people. He admitted that he had occasional depressive thoughts relating to his mother, but, by all accounts, he was managing life well. When Moscovitz met Bella she was sunny, vital and confident. Despite her husband's recent heart surgery Bella believed that they could come through anything together. She had started a business dealing in art and she was doing well. She also worked as magistrate on cases involving children. Here was a puzzle for Moscovitz. *How could four children brought up in the exact same traumatic circumstances land in such vastly different places in life? Why do the Berls and Leahs of the world languish while the Jacks and Bellas cope and even flourish?*

These questions began getting serious attention for the first time in the 1970s when a number of psychologists working at the intersection of child psychiatry and developmental psychology began to investigate the early childhood factors that impeded healthy growth and development. Much of credit goes to Norman Garmezy

(University of Minnesota). While studying children with schizophrenic mothers, Garmezy came across a curious finding. Even in the face of very difficult circumstance, some children could blossom into very decent individuals. Garmezy termed the process as resilience or invulnerability and children as *resilient* or *invulnerable* or *stress-resistant*. It seems that the expression *"resilient"* has become oft-used. The situation can be schematically presented

	Poverty	Prosperity
Competence	Resilient	Advantaged
Incompetence	Vulnerable	Spoiled

The Lotus-in-the-Mud Phenomenon

The foregoing discussion need not create an impression that cases of resilience are limited to successful survivors from the concentration camps. There are other instances in the world context.

In 1989, people of Romania overthrew brutal dictatorship of Nicolae Ceasescu. During his regime, 150000 children were living under appalling conditions in the name of so-called Centre for Family Development. Ceasescu took power in 1965 and his regime required women to have five children by the time they were 45 years of age. They had no access to birth control programmes. Children were malnourished. They slept in dirty cribs. Four children were provided with a single cot. Blankets were soaked in urine and infected with lice. Nearly every ingredient for healthy physical and psychological development was missing.

After the fall of dictatorship, many generous individuals in the developed countries came forward to adopt some of those children. Researchers tracked the

development of these adopted children. A leading researcher compared the development of 46 children who spent between 8 months to 4 ½ years in Romania and were adopted by Canadian parents. They were compared with a group of 46 non-adopted Canadian children. Many adopted children showed significant problems in four specific area:
- IQ was below 85
- Behaviour problems
- Insecure attachment to adopting parents
- Persistence of stereotyped behaviour

However, 2 years after adoption there was significant improvement in physical and psychological conditions. Children who were adopted prior to their 6-month-age were indistinguishable from non-adopted Canadian children. The ability of many children to recover from truly horrific conditions were amazing. Ann Masten, a leading researcher in the area, calls it an *ordinary magic*. According to her, healthy functioning is similar to a rubber band that is stretched but does not break.

There is another incident which is more recent and frightening. On September 11, 2001, the World Trade Center in New York faced terrorist attack and a large number of people were victims of posttraumatic stress disorder (PTSD). The University of California (San Francisco) professor George Bonanno wanted to investigate people's psychological response to such unusual shock.

Bonanno used extensive interviews and was able to break responses down into five main patterns: (1) chronic depression, (2) chronic grief, (3) depressed improved, (4) recovery from grief, and (5) resilient. As indicated by the pattern names, the chronic depression group suffered from pathology both before and after the loss. The chronic grief group functioned well preloss but were paralyzed by grief both immediately after the loss and several years later. The depressed improved group experienced depression before the loss and during the loss, but gradually improved after the loss. The recovery from grief group experienced feelings of grief like yearning, shock, and anxiety that eventually subsided. The resilient group experienced no significant trauma.

The fact that these five patterns emerged did not surprise Bonanno. The real surprise was their relative distribution. over and over again-in natural disasters, after the SARS epidemic following the loss of a child or spouse – Bonanno's longitudinal studies on loss and trauma revealed the same pattern. No matter how bad the trauma, rates of PTSD never exceeded one-third and rates of resilience were always found in at least one-third and never more than two-thirds of the population. It bears repeating that Bonanno was not defining resilience as a lack of feeling or absence of sadness. He used the term "resilient" *to identify people capable of functioning with a sense of core purpose, meaning, and forward momentum in the face of trauma.*

In Indian context, there are also cases of resilient personalities. The resilience phenomenon could otherwise be described as *lotus-in-the-mud phenomenon* (Sahoo 2010). The most fundamental question pertaining resilience concerns the source of resilience.

Source of Resilience

It is fairly difficult to list all possible sources of human resilience. However, a close scrutiny of possible sources may help us to categorize resources into *three* rubrics:
1. **I have (Protective Factors)**
2. **I am (Personality Factors)**
3. **I can (Promotion Factors)**

Protective Factors

The role of protective factors is very important in the development of resilience. The child / youth must have feelings that *I have someone* to count on. Despite poverty / adversity, there is an oasis in the desert of life. The protective factors provide psychological insulation. The person functioning as a protective factor may be one parental figure, or a friend, or a relative, or a teacher, or a neighbor, and so on. It is interestingly found that the child has an empathetic relationship with this protecting individual. If there is disharmony in the family, the child does not report his or her pain / pleasure to parents. If the child receives praise or prize in the school, he/she reports it not to his/her parents, but to the empathetic figure. Similarly, personal agonies are first reported to the protector.

The support of an adult role model buffers the effect of adversity and appears to predict positive outcomes. Such role model is not necessarily a single individual, it could be a small collectivity. High functioning social networks – friends, family, religious and community organizations – may provide protection and support. Werner and Smith (2001) followed nearly seven hundred children growing up in Hawaii with risk factors like poverty, parental discord, and parental stress. Werner and Smith concluded that social factors like supportive relationship function as protective factors.

Two major implications are derived. First, what is important in resilience is the role of a sympathetic adult or institutional agency. Second, such mentoring relationship develops within the framework of everyday experience.

Personality Factors

Theories abound about what produces resilience, but

certain fundamental characteristics seem to set resilient people apart from others. The first characteristic is the capacity to accept and face down reality. In looking hard at reality, we prepare ourselves to act in ways that allow us to endure and survive hardship. A common belief about resilience is that it stems from an optimistic nature. That's true but only as long as such optimism does not distort our sense of reality. In extremely adverse circumstances, rose-coloured thinking can actually spell disaster. In other words, *a blend of realism and optimism is desirable; we may call it realistic optimism or dynamic optimism or functional optimism.*

The ability to see reality is closely linked to the second building block of resilience, the propensity *to make meaning of terrible times*. Generally, people under stress throw up their hands and cry, "How can this be happening to me?" But resilient people devise constructs about their suffering to create some sort of meaning for themselves and others.

The concept is beautifully articulated by Viktor Frankl, an Austrian psychiatrist and Auschwitz concentration camp survivor. In the midst of staggering suffering, Frankl invented *meaning therapy*, a humanistic technique that helps individuals make the kinds of decisions that will create significance in their lives. In his book *Man's Search for Meaning*, Frankl describes the pivotal moment in the camp when he developed meaning therapy. Although he was not sure that he would survive, Frankl imagined himself giving a lecture after the war on the psychology and concentration camp, help outsiders understand what he had been through. He created some concrete goals for himself. In doing so, he succeeded in rising above suffering of the moment. As he put in his book, "We must never forget that we may also find meaning in life even when confronted with a hopeless situation when facing a fate that cannot be changed". Since finding meaning in one's environment is such an important aspect of resilience, it should come as no surprise that the most successful people possess strong value system. Strong value system infuses an individual with meaning because they offer ways to interpret and shape events.

The other building block of resilience is the ability to make do with whatever at hand. Psychologists follow the lead of French anthropologist Levi Strauss in calling this skill *bricolage*. The root of that word is closely tied to the concept of resilience. It literally means "bouncing back". Levi Strauss wrote: "In its old sense, the verb "bricoler" was used with reference to some extraneous movement: a ball rebounding, a dog straying, or a horse swerving from its direct course to avoid an obstacle".

Bricolage in the modern sense can be defined as a kind of inventiveness, an ability to improve solution to a problem without proper or obvious tools or materials. In the concentration camp, for example, resilient inmates knew to pocket pieces of string or wire whenever they found them. The string or wire might later become useful to fix a pair of shoes, which in freezing conditions might make the difference between life and death.

Apart from these main observations, a few other predictors of personal resilience have been identified. In the foregoing discussion, the case of Jack and Bella has been cited. According to Moskovitz's study, Jack and Bella were able to charm the adults and function with self-agency at the Lingfield orphanage, creating a positive feedback loop with the staff and their families that resulted in better and better care. This *ego-resilience* – defined as the capacity to overcome, steer through – was first noted by developmental psychologists, Jack and Jeanne Block in 1968, in a highly regarded longitudinal study documenting the lives of one hundred young adults over more than thirty years. In addition to ego-resilience, the Block study measured a characteristic they called *ego-control*, or the degree to which an individual has the ability to delay gratification in service of future goals. Individuals exhibiting the combination of ego-resilience and ego-control were better able to adapt flexibly to the different circumstances and succeed in the midst of challenges.

Such personality traits are rooted in belief systems that allow one to cognitively reappraise situations and regulate emotions. Social psychologists refer to this as *hardiness* – a system thought, based, broadly on three main tenets: (1) the belief that one can find a meaningful purpose in life, (2) the belief that one can influence one's surroundings and the outcome of events, and (3) the belief that positive and negative experience will lead to learning and growth. Considering this it should come as no surprise that people of faith also report greater degree of resilience.

The role of *religious belief* is a complex issue in the context of resilience. Psychologist Kenneth Pargament has spent the lion share of his academic career investing the links between religion and resilience. Pargament attributes the power of religion to its invocation of the sacred. This connection between religious faith (or, more broadly, a personal spiritual cosmology) and resilience presents an intriguing rejoinder to atheist critic of religious beliefs. While such beliefs may or may not be *true*, they may nonetheless be *adaptive*. That is religious belief persists and thrives, in part, not because it necessarily guarantees persistence of one's soul to the next life, but precisely psychological resilience upon its possessors.

All of these factors are rooted in our beliefs and our

experiences. Whether cultivated through wise mentors, vigorous exercise, access to green space, or a particularly rich relationship with faith, the habits of personal resilience are habits of mind – making them habits we can cultivate and change when armed with the right resources.

This brings us to another less appreciated aspect of personal resilience: the influence of genetics. While the sequencing of human genome in the last decade has provided some useful information regarding genetic triggers, the current research has focused the effectiveness of tools that complement other forms of intervention for promoting resilience.

Promoting Factors

There are quite a few mechanisms that can be used as intervention to promise resilience. Yet one tool is portable, teachable, free and it's been on the market for more than two thousand years. It is meditation.

Researchers who study mindfulness and attention often conceive our emotions differently. In their view, emotions are not things that happen to us. Rather they exist – metaphorically, of course – as a kind of psychic currency, held in reserve. When we waste the reserve – giving over our attention to every single distraction from the outside environment – it dwindles down into an empty account, and we are left feeling fatigued or worse, in a downward spiral of negative affects like anger and greed. With practice, on the other hand, we can train ourselves to spend judiciously, keeping us from draining our emotional coffers.

Mindfulness meditation training is the tool that lets us do so. It allows us to take more intentional control over our emotions. Some of the training is drawn from Buddhism. These tools of meditation, mindfulness, and increasing awareness have been proven to aid in resilience training. Richard Davidson, the leading light in the area of neuroscience, opines that the eastern tradition in meditation is even effective in neuroplasticity – the process of rewiring (changing) the brain.

There are many systems of meditation. Meditation experts often refer to two different styles: focused-attention and open monitoring. Focused-attention meditation maintains attention on a specific object of concentration. When thoughts and sensation arise, the mind allows them to pass without clinging to them and then brings itself back to focus on the chosen object.

In open monitoring, on the other hand, the object of focus recedes, and a sustained awareness of all sensory experience is cultivated. Open monitoring is characterized by an open, present, and nonjudgmental awareness of stimuli in the environment.

There is a third type of mediation that plays pivotal role in personal resilience. It is often called "loving kindness" or a practice of compassionate meditation. This is the technique of cultivating greater empathy through meditation. Such practices produce significant activity in the insula – a region near the frontal portion of the brain that plays a key role in bodily representations of emotion. In this practice, the mediator first focuses on loved ones and then expands the focus of compassion to towards all beings. Neuroscientist Davidson appreciates its role in altering our brain chemistry.

Finally, it is important to recognize that positivity of psychological resilience is not limited to the triumph over adversity. The gains are not confined to getting around the problem of post-traumatic stress disorder (PTSD). Rather the resilience may bring the benefits of *post-traumatic growth*. It has been shown that a number of people experience growth following traumatic events. They may change their lifestyles in the positive direction. They may give up smoking, renew family harmony and do many other prosocial activities. In view of these positive expectations, researchers are now gravitating from the study of PTSD to the exploration of *PTG (Post-traumatic growth)*.

■

Pandemic and Rebuilding of Life

The horror and terror generated by COVID 19 pandemic has raised a fundamental question: What would be the ultimate outcome of corona virus real life trauma? It is true that the real impact would surface in course of time. In order to assess the impact of a big event, we need a time gap. The impact of French Revolution could be assessed only after the gap of a few decades. People in general and social and behavioural scientists in particular would be able to assess the impact. It is likely that social and behavioural scientists have already initiated their search process and the results of their investigation are awaited.

Despite such human guessing and waiting, it is possible to form hunches and hypotheses. In the past the human tragedy of various dimensions and forms have struck the world. Traumas of various kinds (personal tragedies in form of deadly diseases such as cancer, HIV & SARS, natural catastrophes such as cycles, super cyclone, earthquake, volcanoes, civil wars, terrorists attack) have afflicted mankind. Men of science have intensively studied the impacts with a view to staging preparedness for future threats.

The outcome of the search process in the past has generated a number of immensely useful take aways.

Post-Traumatic Stress Disorder (PTSD)

In recent years PTSD (post-traumatic stress disorder) has become an oft-used term in our contemporary life. A person or a child may experience trauma at the personal level (losing parents at an early age, having a deadly disease, being caught in a fire tragedy, and so on). The individual may also encounter trauma as a member of a bigger group as in calamities of floods hurricanes, super cyclone, earthquake and volcanic eruptions. The victims of such tragedies are likely to lose their psychological balance and develop behavioural disorders.

The trauma produces severe stress resulting in a number of mental and behaviour disorders. The **PTSD (Post-Traumatic Stress Disorder)** induces intense form of fear and then the individual experiences anger. Since the person is dumbstruck, the perception of external reality is severely lowered. After a month or so, conditions slightly improve yet the person stays in a confused state and does not take initiative for social contact.

Although normalcy is restored after one month in some cases, severity of negative symptoms increases in many persons. The second phase (next six months) is a period of *numbness*. The feeling of afflicted persons is severely restricted. During this numbing period, there are several strange symptoms. The individual prefers social isolation. The manifested symptoms are of three types. First, individuals stay hyper vigilant. The sound of a dropping leaf from the tree scares the person. The person is unnecessarily irritable. Depression and anxiety are displayed.

Apart from intense negative emotion (anger, fear and depression), some *intrusive* symptoms are shown. Persons with PTSD experience disturbed sleep, gets up from the bed and stays awake. The native flashbacks disturb the individual. Without apparent reason the person experiences guilt: "Why did it happen to me. If it happened to me; it could happen to any one in this world".

The third type of symptom is social apathy. The person does not experience *empathy*, does not feel sad when someone is miserable and does not feel happy at the happiness of others.

On the whole the trauma produces symptoms that make the victims dysfunctional. Although psychologists have identified the causal factors at the deeper levels of consciousness, these are beyond the scope of present discussion. The alleviation of the symptoms and treatment require psychiatric help. The most surprising element of PTSD is the observation that all people subjected to trauma don't show psychological break-downs. A sizable section shows positive changes following trauma called Post Traumatic Growth (PTG).

Post-Traumatic Growth (PTG)

It is quite surprising that many people find meaningful life lessons, a renewed appreciation for life and increased feeling of personal strength as a result of traumatic experiences. In contrast to the negative outcomes that characterize post-traumatic stress disorder (PTSD), positive outcomes have been referred to as **post-traumatic growth (PTG)**. It is also interesting to observe that almost one-third of the victims of trauma display PTG. Sociologists and psychologists have observed victims of Hitler's concentration camps, victims of several civil wars, the afflicted persons of terrorists' attack on World Trade Center during September of 2001 and victims of all sorts of natural calamities. They have concluded that two-third of the victims show negativity while one-third of the afflicted display PTG.

Initially traumatic experiences are frightening and disorienting. Over time, some people learn deeper lessons about themselves and about life. These lessons have the potential to enhance individual's understanding of themselves, their relationships, and their priorities. These lessons contribute to more effective coping and adjustment.

Positive changes are manifest in *three* domains of life. There are changes in individual's perception. Individuals experience an increased feeling of personal strength, confidence and self-reliance. They develop a greater appreciation of the fragility of life including one's own.

There are remarkable changes in relationship. Persons feel closer ties to family. They give up bad habits such as smoking and drinking. They make greater emotional disclosure and feelings of closeness to others. They display greater compassion for others and more willingness to help others.

More importantly *changes in life priorities* are manifest. They experience greater clarity about what is important in life. A deeper and often spiritual sense of the meaning in life develops. A new commitment to take life easier takes shape. In addition, individuals show less concern with acquiring material possessions, money and social status.

Explanations for positive growth through trauma have drawn on the work of existential psychologist Viktor Frankl (1959/1976). Frankl, the Auschwitz death-camp survivor, argues that a **"will to meaning"** is a basic motivating force in people's lives. People, according to him, seek a sense of purpose, meaning and a direction to sustain them through life's journey. The sense of meaning helps people to interpret trauma-based losses, it also helps people to renew life with new interpretation. Thus, human capacity to prevail over adversity generates the possibility of growth through trauma.

Yet, the fundamental question remains: **Which of the victim segments would experience PTG?** Fortunately, empirical studies of the past, including some experimentally controlled studies. Provide scientific answers.

Studies of Mortality Reminders

The systematic investigation of the effects of trauma and its effects on producing PTSD vis-à-vis PTG has taken various forms. A number of investigators have examined the impact of real-life traumas such as personal trauma (loss of parents at an early age, terminal diseases), natural calamities and global tragedies such as civil wars and terrorists attack (attack on World Trade Centre). The observation and analysis of such events have provided some hunches and hypotheses that have been further verified through systematic experiments.

It appears that *three* elements of trauma generate the possibility of PTG. First, the time factor is important. The experience of trauma needs to be relatively *durable*. A temporary and short-lived traumatic experience may stay for a while and goes away. It many not induce any positive change. Second, the feeling associated with trauma may be very *intense* to produce PTG. Third, the crucial element which induces PTG is not just the death–related thoughts, it is *death reflection*. The death reflection prompts the individual to review his/her life, to search for meaning and accentuate religious/spiritual orientation of life.

The scientific proofs in favor of PTG (changes in the direction of intrinsic motivation and values) may briefly be described. In one study, researchers attempted to create *awareness of death* by manipulating what is known as **mortality salience**. This involved brief exposure to death – related scenes (e.g., funeral homes, dead bodies, etc.). A common procedure involved simply asking participants of the study to write down their thoughts, feelings and emotions when thinking about their own death. Following such experience, participants are asked to indicate their attitudes, values and goals. It is interesting to note that participants, compared to their pre-exposure session or control group participants, show greater shifts to material values and possessions. For example, they now aspire for a better car, more luxurious house, higher salary and larger recreation facility. It is interpreted that the mortality reminders persuade them to make use of a culture-given protection blanket in the form of extrinsic support system (money and materials).

In contrast, another study was directed to generate vicarious death reflections manipulation that paralleled the essential features of near-death experience. Participants in the near-death condition were asked to imagine that they are trapped in apartment fire-tragedy. They struggled to escape but failed. With such a manipulation, the findings indicated a shift towards intrinsic values (kindness, compassion and spirituality).

Take-Aways

Results of both studies suggest that PTG occurs with confronting an actual life-threatening experience. Such conditions increase awareness of life's ulterior aims. Death reflection needs to occur over some period of time rather than being a quick consideration that will most likely produce defensive reactions (longing for money and materials). Second, thinking about mortality needs to prompt life review in which death is incorporated into life and accepted, rather than denied. Third, it seems important that death reflection includes consideration of how friends and family would respond to one's own death. These propositions have been amply supported by many empirical studies including the survey of earthquakes victims of North Bridge catastrophe in California in the year 1994.

■

Finding Silver Lining in a Cloud

Looking at the bright side is a positive mindset. However, it is not only celebrating the present and the past, but anticipating a bright future. Being optimistic involves a choice about how you see the world. It doesn't mean denying the negative or avoiding all uncomfortable information. It also doesn't mean constantly trying to control situations that cannot be controlled. Indeed, research shows that optimists are more, or less, vigilant of risks and threats.

Big Optimism versus Small Optimism

One may ordinarily think that optimism as a trait is self-consistent; one who is optimistic about small events is also optimistic about big events. This is not necessarily true. A person may have small optimism in the sense he or she thinks it possible to complete his or her day's work in time. Yet, the person may not be confident of fulfilling his or her life goals (the pat of bigger optimism). Similarly, an individual may possess big optimism in the sense that he or she considers himself/herself capable of achieving bigger objectives. Yet the individual may not be sure of completing day-to-day mundane activities. However, it is difficult to ascertain the degree of linkage between small optimism and big optimism.

Explanatory Styles

Martin Seligman, the renowned positive psychologist, has offered an interesting cognitive principle underlying optimism. According to Seligman, every person asks three fundamental questions while encountering a good situation or a bad situation. The modality of their answers determines their optimistic versus pessimistic style.

When people encounter negative (bad) events, they ask three fundamental questions: Who is responsible? How long would this effect stay? How pervasive would be the effect? The answer to the first question ranges from "me totally" to "other persons or outside circumstances completely". If people blame themselves completely for the bad event (an internal attribution), the depression and pessimism would be intense. On the contrary, explaining bad events in terms of external factors would reduce the intensity of depression/pessimism. In other words, internal attribution to explain bad events would bring pessimism whereas external attributions for explaining bad events would bring optimism.

Furthermore, people may have the tendency to explain bad (negative) events in terms of stable factors. They may consider bad events as permanent. This will augment pessimism. In contrast, other category of people many consider bad events as temporary. This is likely to reduce pessimism. In other words, stable attribution brings pessimism and unstable attribution induces optimism. The other dimension involves global versus specific attribution. When a bad event happens, an individual may spill over the effect to other areas of life. (e.g., My friend has betrayed me; what is the guarantee that my boss would take cognizance of my merit? This is generalization from social domain to work domain). In contrast, another individual may employ specific attribution in the context of bad events. For example, a person may get his hand fractured because of an accident. Yet the person may use specific attribution: I can no longer work with my hands to operate a machine, but I can proofread in a press using my eyes. Thus, generalization is checked and spilling over is avoided. Thus, global (general) attribution spreads pessimism and specificity induces optimism in the context of bad events.

How do optimists explain positive (good) events? For optimism and adaptation, people need to explain positive events in terms of three P^s (Personal, Permanent, and Pervasive). Whenever good events happen, they may think of *personal* involvement (e.g., I have at least made the guest-contact in our annual function). They also need to stretch the effect over bone. Considering the effect *permanent*, they find it useful to prolong good feeling. The effect is also viewed as *pervasive* spilling the positive effects to many areas of their lives. The good things happening at home may be discussed in the workplace. Similarly positive moods generated in the workplace may be shared with family members. This kind of generalization would spread optimism.

In sum, an optimistic approach involves explaining negative events in terms of external, unstable and specific factors. In contrast, the approach views positive events in personal (internal), permanent (stable) and pervasive (global) terms.

Fostering Optimism

In view of several benefits of optimism, psychologists and counsellors have advised people to cultivate optimism. There are several routes to the goal of building optimism.

The Best Possible Selves Exercise. The University of

Missouri-Columbia professor Laura King pioneered the first ever systematic intervention of optimism. She asked participants to visit her laboratory for four consecutive days. On each day they were instructed to spend twenty minutes writing a narrative description of their "best possible future selves". Basically this is a mental exercise in which you visualize the best possible future for yourself in multiple domains of life. For example, a twenty-five-year-old young man might imagine that in ten years, he will have a managerial job, would get married, settle for family and would provide good education to his children. This is essentially his fantasy of what his life might be like if all his dreams were realized. Then again, perhaps the term *fantasy* is poorly chosen, in as much as it implies that the vision of his life is only a fanciful farfetched daydream. To the contrary, this exercise involves considering your most important, deeply held goals and picturing that they will be achieved. Laura King found that people who wrote about their visions for twenty minutes per day over several days, relative to those who wrote about other topics, were more likely to show immediate increases in positive moods to be happier several weeks later, and even to report fewer physical ailments several month thence.

The Best Possible Selves exercise turned out to be a potent intervention. Lyubomirsky applied it in laboratory. She instructed participants to do just one writing session in the lab, and then urged them to continue the writing session at home, as often and for as long as they wished, over four weeks. As expected, participants who engaged in the Best Possible Selves exercise showed a significant lift in their positive mood.

In addition to the Best Possible Selves strategy, there are other ways to tap optimistic thinking. The strategies do work for several reasons. First, optimistic thoughts can be *self-fulfilling* properties. When you are confident that you will be able to achieve your lifelong goals, you will invest efforts in reaching those goals. Another important way that optimistic thinking enhances well-being is that it prompts us to engage in active and effective coping. Furthermore, optimistic thinking promotes positive moods, vitality and high morale.

Best Possible Selves diary. Best Possible Selves diary method is very useful. To try it out, sit in a quiet place, and take twenty to thirty minutes to think about what you expect your life will be one, five, or ten years from now. Visualize a future for yourself in which everything has turned out the way you wanted. The writing exercise in a sense puts your optimistic "muscles" into practice.

Goals and subgoals diary. A twist on the Best Possible Selves diary is that as part of developing hopeful thinking, you identify your long-range goals and break them into subgoals. For example, during the first session of your journal writing, you could describe how five years from now you will be owner of your own business. In subsequent sessions you could write about step you would take to fulfil your main goal.

Identify barrier thoughts. Another strategy to increase optimistic thinking involves identifying automatic negative thoughts. For example, you might put a small coin in a jar each time you have a pessimistic thought. Then try to replace that thought with a more favourable point of view.

Making Optimistic Habit

Essentially, all optimism strategies involve the exercise of construing the world with a more positive and charitable perspective, and many entail considering the silver lining in the cloud, identifying the door that opens. It takes hard work and a great deal of practice to accomplish effectively, but if you can persist in these strategies until they become habitual the benefits would be immense. Some optimists may be born that way, but scores of optimists are made with practice.

The psychologist Lee Ross: "Optimism is not about providing a recipe for self-deception. The world can be a horrible, cruel place, and at the same time it can be wonderful and abundant. These are both truths. There is not a halfway point, there is only choosing which truth to put in your personal foreground."

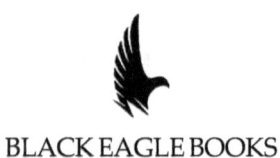

BLACK EAGLE BOOKS

www.blackeaglebooks.org
info@blackeaglebooks.org

Black Eagle Books, an independent publisher, was founded as a nonprofit organization in April, 2019. It is our mission to connect and engage the Indian diaspora and the world at large with the best of works of world literature published on a collaborative platform, with special emphasis on foregrounding Contemporary Classics and New Writing.

www.ingramcontent.com/pod-product-compliance
Lightning Source LLC
Chambersburg PA
CBHW020532080526
44583CB00013B/831